Chro
and the T

Chronic Illness
and the Twelve Steps
A Practical Approach to Spiritual Resilience

MARTHA CLEVELAND, PH.D.

1949-1999
HAZELDEN

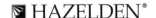

HAZELDEN®

INFORMATION & EDUCATIONAL SERVICES

Hazelden
Center City, Minnesota 55012-0176
1-800-328-0094
1-651-213-4590 (Fax)
www.hazelden.org

(Formerly titled *The Twelve Step Response to Chronic Illness and Disability: Recovering Joy in Life* and *Living Well: A Twelve-Step Response to Chronic Illness and Disability*)
First published 1988 by Hazelden
Printed in the United States of America

Library of Congress Cataloging-in-Publication Data

Cleveland, Martha.
    [Twelve step response to chronic illness and disability]
    Chronic illness and the twelve steps : a practical approach to
spiritual resilience / Martha Cleveland.
        p.   cm.
    Includes bibliographical references and index.
    ISBN 1-56838-347-9
    1. Chronic diseases—Psychological aspects. 2. Twelve-step
programs. I. Title.
RC108.C54   1999
616'.044'019—dc21
                                                                            99-16590
                                                                            CIP

              03 02 01 00 99   6 5 4 3 2 1

Editor's note

The Twelve Steps are reprinted and adapted with permission of Alcoholics Anonymous World Services, Inc. Permission to reprint and adapt the Twelve Steps does not mean that AA has reviewed or approved the contents of this publication, or that AA necessarily agrees with the views expressed herein. AA is a program of recovery from alcoholism *only*—use of the Twelve Steps in connection with programs and activities which are patterned after AA, but which address other problems, or in any other non-AA context, does not imply otherwise.

The vignettes in this book are composites based on the experiences of chronically ill and disabled people. Any resemblance to actual persons, living or dead, or specific situations, is entirely coincidental.

Cover design by David Spohn
Interior design by Donna Burch
Typesetting by Stanton Publication Services, Inc.

Note to the Reader

Clarification of terms: Within the text of this book, "Higher Power" and "spiritual resources" are meant to be interchangeable. Both terms refer to whatever gives us strength, hope, and serenity and enhances our humanity. "Disabled/disability" and "physically challenged" are also used interchangeably. Either term means any condition that limits physical function.

M. C.

To my husband, Walter, and my children, Mark, Jayne, and David—who have unfailingly and lovingly supported me, all of our time together.

Contents

Preface

This book was first published in 1988 under the title *The Twelve Step Response to Chronic Illness and Disability.* Its true mission was expressed in its original subtitle, "Recovering Joy in Life." Since then, I have heard from many people that the premise of the book is true. Those of us with chronic illnesses or disabilities often have a great deal of emotional pain with which we struggle. The Twelve Step program has proven to be an incredibly powerful tool for releasing that pain and building a strong and healthy life. As spiritual life strengthens, physical life becomes more satisfying and serene.

A man at a party once said to me, "My mother is eighty and her bones are breaking down from osteoporosis. She has a copy of your book on the table by her chair, and she has used it so much that it's almost in tatters." My heart filled with concern and care for this gallant woman, and of course I sent her a new copy. In another instance, a social worker from New York asked for permission to use the material in the workshops she presents for professionals who work with chronically ill or disabled people. I also heard from a man who belongs to a Disabilities Anonymous group that uses the book as a recovery guide. It is being used as the basis for support groups on the Internet as well. Whether it's an individual, or a teacher, or a group; whether it is through personal interaction or through the miracles of technology; for people with chronic illnesses or disabilities, following the Twelve Step program leads to a better life.

In the last dozen years there have been many medical and social changes. The explosion of AIDS has led to an emphasis on understanding the immune response and its effect on the body. We have more effective anti-inflammatory drugs, new antidepressants and antipsychotics, and drugs to help people with Parkinson's disease. We have a far better understanding of the connection between lifestyle and heart disease and the management of high blood pressure. We are able to detect and treat many more cancers than in the past. There are now miraculous prostheses for amputees, much improved products for ostomy patients, and more realistic cosmetic aids for hair and dental loss. The list goes on and on, and new breakthroughs are always around the corner.

Socially, there have been changes too. In 1990, Congress passed the Americans with Disabilities Act. This has led to better physical access and financial support for persons who are physically or emotionally challenged. As a whole, our society has a much improved sensitivity to, and awareness of, individual disability. The birth of the Internet has led to an international forum where people with all kinds of chronic illness and physical challenges can gather information. There are also mailing lists and chat rooms where people can support each other and share information.

But at the same time that medical, social, and technological changes lead us into the new millennium with much hope, each individual person whose life has been challenged by a chronic illness or some kind of disability must live today and tomorrow, one day at a time. There is no magic cure for the emotional pain we carry; and, as I did so many years ago, each of us must find his or her own way.

Acknowledgments

I want to thank Corrine Casanova, my editor, for her unfailing availability, courtesy, enthusiasm, and encouragement during this revision. I also want to thank the people who have read, and used, the earlier edition of the book. Knowing that it has been useful to valiant people is, for me, a gift beyond price. Finally, I want to thank my own errant immune system without whose relentless unpredictability I might never have found this way to live.

Joy Will Come in the Morning

I was thirty-three years old when I first got really sick. I felt exhausted and depressed, with aching joints and fingernails that kept splitting and peeling off. My body had continual itchy rashes that no antihistamine or lotion could relieve. My blood profile showed that something was wrong, but none of the doctors could say exactly what it was. Then I lost my hair. All of it. Every single hair on my body fell out. They called it Alopecia Universalis. I was grotesque, a freak. One psychiatrist wanted to take my picture for a textbook. I was so ashamed, anxious, and insecure that I almost let him. I shudder to think how I would have felt today, knowing that for generations to come medical students would see me as a physical aberration.

I was told that there was no remedy. The doctors felt that it was probably due to emotional stress. They told me to relax. I cried a lot, raged some, felt helpless, hopeless, alone, and terrified. My days buzzed with anxiety; my nights were filled with visions of screaming and suffocating. But my husband and children needed me, and my friends kept calling, so I put on an awful wig and crept back into life. Two years later, my hair came back, but my blood counts remained abnormal and life was never to be the same.

As I grew older, my hair fell out again, and then again,

Introduction

and still no help was available. Not only was there no medical aid, but my doctors were unable to give me any emotional support. They didn't know how to fix my body and weren't trained to deal with my soul. Fortunately, today there is an increasing acknowledgment in the medical field that bodies, psyches, and souls are intertwined.

When I was fifty, I finally went to a well-known rheumatologist (a specialist in muscle and joint disease) who said, "Your problem isn't stress, not basically anyway; your body just doesn't work right. You've got a physical problem. I can tell you what's wrong, but I can't do anything for you. There's something haywire with your immune system, and we don't know much about immune systems. Someday we'll be able to treat people like you with something, much like we treat diabetics today. It probably won't kill you, and it's not your fault." That was nearly twenty years ago. I cried once more, but this time with relief and gratitude. Then I began the long road to understanding how to live with a chronic illness.

Today I would have been diagnosed with a form of lupus (an autoimmune disease). Having a "legitimate" diagnosis would have been helpful as I went on to develop other chronic inflammatory conditions such as Sjogren's Syndrome and atopic dermatitis. But chances are, if I would have had a "legitimate" diagnosis, I would have never searched for my own solutions and would never have found the Twelve Steps (part of the Alcoholics Anonymous recovery program).

In his book *Living with a Chronic Illness*, Daniel Anderson, Ph.D., tells us that of all the health care problems in the United States today, nearly 80 percent relate to chronic illness or disability. There are a lot of us out there. While the medical community helps manage our acute episodes, it is not structured to give us the kind of support we need to last the rest of our lives. Whether our condition is a physical problem that life has dealt us, such as chronic heart disease, a nervous system disorder, cancer, diabetes, hepatitis, an autoimmune disease or AIDS; or whether it is a major emotional impairment such as schizophrenia or a manic-depressive disorder, we sometimes feel that our situation is unbearable.

How we deal with the unbearable is largely our choice. Unfortunately, too often our response creates as much stress as the disease or physical challenge itself. In our confusion, fear, and anger, we may react in ways that limit us and leave us living diminished lives. But we can change this. While we can't alter the fact that our chronic illness or disability may never be healed, we can learn to live in a way that reduces the stress on ourselves and those around us. We can stop making our physical problems worse and help ourselves to become happier, more productive people.

I believe that most people with chronic illness or disability also suffer from intense and chronic emotional pain. This pain equals and often surpasses the physical pain or physical challenge caused by our condition. We may feel lonely, angry, depressed, or hopeless. Feelings of isolation and powerlessness begin to set the boundaries of our lives. In our emotional pain, we may reduce our involvement with family, friends, and co-workers. Then people tell us that our emotional struggles can make our chronic condition worse; so we add to our load, blaming ourselves for not relaxing and accepting things as they are. In our heart of hearts, we know that we have only this one life to live, and we yearn to become the very most we can be in the time we have. For many of us, it is terribly hard to remember that. Whatever our physical or mental limitations, we are incomparable individuals who can make a unique contribution to our world. While we can't control the reality of our illness or disability, we *can* choose how to respond emotionally and spiritually to that reality.

The Alcoholics Anonymous (AA) recovery program offers a unique method we can use to triumph over our emotional pain—a method we will explore in this book. AA is a program originally developed by alcoholics for alcoholics to help themselves and each other recover from their self-destructive behavior. It is now a worldwide organization that touches millions of lives. The core of AA is the Twelve Steps, which can be "worked" one day at a time. Those alcoholics (and now many other struggling people) who work the program by studying, interpreting, and integrating its philosophy into their lives are "in recovery." This recovery process is a lifetime commitment.

The Twelve Step program is spiritual, based on action coming from love. In countries all around the world it has been the most effective method of dealing with alcoholism. In addition to being used in the treatment of alcoholics, it is now being used to treat other conditions such as sexual addiction, eating disorders, gambling, and addiction to drugs other than alcohol. The belief that underlies this book is that it can also be effective in overcoming the emotional pain connected with chronic illness and disability.

The Twelve Steps are directed toward spiritual growth. If we adapt this program to our unique situations and apply its principles to our individual lives, we can outmaneuver the effects of our physical illness with spiritual wellness. This is not an easy process. It demands serious commitment and a willingness to change our behaviors as well as our belief systems. But if we truly trust in the recovery process, things do change. Our feelings of depression and isolation lift as we find a spiritual common ground with others who share our experience. Our hatred of powerlessness changes as we learn to truly accept, rather than simply accommodate, the unmanageability of our bodies. We transform powerlessness into a tool that helps us find peace in our lives. No matter what our physical or mental limitations, we can work toward a fulfilled life, one lived without fear, shame, or loneliness and supported by love, serenity, and joy.

It is the premise of this book that while we do not have ultimate control over our bodies, we absolutely do have control over the fulfillment of our spiritual potential. We can get beyond the effects of the cultural definitions that are placed on us and that we often accept. In this process our spirits will become flexible and strong. We will finally learn to live through the grace that is at the center of every human being.

It is my hope that this book will help people who live

with chronic illness or some type of physical disability. In the first three chapters, I have explained the problem as I have come to see it through my own experience and while working with others. Chapters 4 through 13 take us through the Twelve Steps of AA, redefined here so each Step becomes especially meaningful to us. Chapter 14 is a hopeful prophecy, describing what the outcome of our commitment to spiritual wellness can be. Finally, I have included lists of the Twelve Steps, the Serenity Prayer, daily meditations, and information about contacting mutual aid groups.

An old African American spiritual tells us, "Weeping may endure for a night, but joy will come in the morning." Together we can find that morning.

CHAPTER ONE

"Our Wound Is the Place . . ."

Our wound is the place where our soul finds entry into us. The calamity that strikes may be our call to spiritual fulfillment.
—Ernest Lawrence Rossi

In the beginning there were two perfect people—a man named Adam and a woman named Eve. They glowed with health and beauty as they surrounded themselves in a garden full of light, trees, and flowers. The serpent, whose name was Reality, lay coiled behind a rock, unseen and unheeded. After a while, Reality became tired of being ignored and slid through time and the woods into another garden.

Things were very different here in this new garden. The sun was bright, trees grew, and flowers bloomed, but clouds dotted the blue sky and a few weeds sprouted among the blossoms. The people were different too. Many looked strong and healthy, but some were bent, some blind, some sat in wheelchairs, and some stood tall with faces that showed pain and suffering. This garden was Reality's home.

Perhaps it is from these conflicting images that we look at our world. We know where Reality lives, but we act as if Reality doesn't exist. We honor beauty and reject imperfection. We have beauty pageants and may try to convince ourselves that a contestant's talents are important in the judging. But most of us know that what wins is the perfect face, the shiny hair, the slender legs, and the sexy body in a bathing suit. Our television personalities and politicians—people who help shape the way we view our world—are painted, coiffed, sprayed, and color-coded to one-dimensional perfection. It's easy for us to blame advertising and the media, but they only offer what many of us want so badly ourselves: physical and mental perfection. We tell ourselves that if we look well-groomed and healthy and don't show or talk about afflictions, then we will be good, worthwhile people who belong. The tragedy here is that this leaves a society of mostly imperfect people trying to become perfect. What about those of us who are not perfect, who don't glow with health and beauty, who are in some significant way different? As children, most of us learn that to have a physical imperfection is not "normal." To be ill or injured is acceptable only if it heals quickly, doesn't leave scar tissue, and we cry about it as little as possible. Children born with a physical or mental differentness are taught while they are still very young to hide or disguise this difference. As this lesson sinks in, they also learn to be ashamed of their disability.

Those of us who develop chronic illness or disability later in life have also learned these lessons. All our lives we may have been taught not to stare and that we should ignore another's difference. When we become afflicted, we feel as though we are joining a group of people who are somehow undesirable and outside the normal boundaries of society. We become defined by our wound, illness, or disability, and many of us come to believe that definition. We use up our emotional energies in our struggle to prove ourselves to others, to "pass," pretend, or in some other way be just like everyone else. In this struggle to hide or reject our differentness, we forget that it is part of us. If we reject it, we end up rejecting an integral part of our self. We damage our souls even more than our illness damages our bodies.

From Darkness to Light

Our culture loses much by refusing to honor the darker things in life. Wounds and shadows can offer great gifts. For one thing, they offer balance; they allow us to see life whole. Most of life's meaning is defined in terms of contrasts. We can't really experience light unless we have known darkness; we don't know what sweet is until we taste sour. When we fill a white bowl with red petunias, the red becomes more brilliant, the white clearer. Joy often rises from sadness, and love seems more precious when we know the violence of hate.

Wise people throughout the ages have written that we can't fully live life until we have accepted our own mortality. How often, when our lives or the lives of our loved ones are threatened, do we yearn for the treasure of a quiet walk, a few minutes in a favorite chair with the cat curled in our lap, an uneventful evening of TV, or a hot bath and a good book? Time and time again we hear from terminally ill people that in knowing they are going to lose life, they find its meaning and cherish each moment of the time that they have left. The same insight comes to many of us who become chronically ill or disabled. The loss of complete health or full physical function shakes us up, and our priorities settle in a different order. As we question our future, we learn to live more completely in the present. We give and take from life without assuming there will be a tomorrow and another tomorrow. We stop taking life for granted and start noticing it.

Also, accepting and understanding wounds and shadows release us from fear. When we are able to live openly with the imperfections of ourselves and others, these imperfections become familiar companions. They are no longer frightening ghosts to be hidden or denied. How freeing it would be to say, "I have cancer," or "I shake because I have Parkinson's disease," rather than to make up excuses about baldness or fatigue or a trembling hand. How much more comfortable it would be to say, "Can I help you?" to the woman in a wheelchair who is trying to reach an item on the store shelf, rather than to hold back, afraid to hurt her feelings or anger her. When we deny our illnesses or disabilities by pretending they don't exist, we make them shameful and give them power over ourselves and others. Only recognizing and accepting them can free us from our fear.

Finally, physical and emotional wounds offer a place for our souls to enter. This doesn't mean that people without illnesses or disabilities are without souls. But without facing the realities of impairment, it's easier to deny spiritual development and expend energy chasing physical perfection. How often we hear someone who has faced, or is facing, a serious crisis say, "It's awful, but I've learned about what's important in life and have seen how to make life better for me." Wayne Muller, in a wonderful spiritual guide called *How, Then, Shall We Live?* says:

> This is what I have learned: Within the sorrow [within our wound] here is grace. When we come close to things that break us down, we touch those things that break us open. And in breaking open, we uncover our true nature.

Psychology tells us that changes in life's circumstances bring about change in people. When lives are disrupted, people have to be different to adapt to the new situation. When we are disabled or chronically ill, we are faced with a challenge: How are we going to handle this?

Our Spirits Are Still Ours

For those of us who live with chronic illness or disability, the challenge is clear. Our bodies are no longer predictable, our trust in our physical self is shaken, and nature seems out of control. But our spirit is still ours and always will be. Spiritual fulfillment can be our goal. Our souls can support and guide us on whatever path our bodies take.

It's very hard to define individual human spirituality. Just when we think we have come up with an explanation, some part of it eludes us. Some people believe in an external, personal God, a force outside of themselves. For them, spiritual growth and fulfillment come through a strengthening relationship with this God. Others recognize an impersonal Power or Force greater than themselves to which they can turn for help as they struggle with their lives. Still others find spiritual development in their individual integrity and their interaction with the universe. Whatever approach they take, people reach spiritual fulfillment by attending to and expanding the life force within them.

Our spirituality is our essence, our energy toward life. To grow spiritually is to use that energy in a positive way, so that both our own lives and the lives of those around us are enriched. M. Scott Peck, in *The Road Less Traveled*, tells us that love is the will to extend ourselves for the purpose of nurturing our own or someone else's spiritual growth. So when we commit ourselves to spiritual growth, we commit ourselves to love. This is a lifelong process. There is never a point where we graduate to some higher state of permanent fulfillment. But if we dedicate ourselves to spiritual growth, and if we truly believe in the potential of our spirit, we will come to be full of life and at peace within that fullness.

When we are disabled or chronically ill, our spirit is tested. It can be crushed, leading us to rage, desperation, or despair. Or it can be challenged, leading us to love, acceptance, and serenity. The choice is up to each one of us. Even if our physical condition seems out of control, we can choose how to react to our illness or disability. We can see it as a threat or as a challenge. We can become shriveled, mean, with eyes always looking inward. Or we can reach out, becoming all that we can be with everything we have. In *The Secret Garden*, a beautiful book about overcoming illness and grief, the old gardener tells the children that thistles can't grow where roses are cultivated—and this is true. We can let our thistles grow, or we can choose to nurture roses.

CHAPTER TWO

Who's Challenged?

So who's challenged? The answer is—anyone. Anyone at any moment may become challenged by disease, a freak accident, a birth defect, the wrong combination of genes, or the physical or mental breakdowns that come with aging. Our challenged group contains people of both sexes and people of all ages. Black, white, Asian, Christian, Jewish, Muslim, agnostic or atheist, rich or poor—none of this matters. Who you are or where you came from is irrelevant. If the challenge comes, it's yours regardless.

Some of us are challenged by a disability that shows: It is clear for the world to see.

Senator Daniel Inouye of Hawaii makes no attempt to hide his missing arm. My blind mother feels her way across an unfamiliar room with her cane extended to warn her of obstacles. A young male paraplegic maneuvers his wheelchair through a crowded aisle in Kmart. An acquaintance fiddles with her hearing aid. The child in front of you turns her head, and you may be shocked to see that she has Down's syndrome.

Many others walk with hidden illness.

The woman next to you in the grocery checkout line has cancer in her stomach. There is no way you can know. Your business associate quietly takes his blood pressure medication at lunch and studies the menu for low-salt, low-fat food. He doesn't comment, and no one notices. A recovering alcoholic lawyer nurses a glass of ginger ale at a cocktail party. The older woman next to you at the movies shifts in her seat as she tries to still the raging arthritis in her hip. Her quick frown seems meaningless.

In addition to those who carry illness or disability there are all the others who love and care for them.

The woman in the grocery checkout line has a cancer that is not only hers, but her family's. Her husband wonders how he can support her and take care of their home while she is ill from chemotherapy. Her children watch her, afraid she will die and leave them. All of them think about how her illness means putting aside their own needs in life. The young paraplegic's mother worries that he won't marry and will have a lonely life. His father is afraid that his son will never feel like a man. His girlfriend is caught between her love for him and her grief in giving up her dream of a strong and healthy husband. The wife of the recovering alcoholic lawyer secretly watches him at the party, pushing aside her fear that he might drink again.

These people are challenged too.

When people are struck with chronic illness or disability, they tend to feel powerless. But for family and friends, the situation is much different. In their eyes, from the moment of onset, the person with the illness or disability gains great power. Family life becomes organized around the needs and limitations of the chronically ill or disabled person. When a fifteen-year-old boy comes home from the rehab hospital as a paraplegic, the entire structure of the house has to be changed. Ramps are built, doors are widened, and bedrooms are rearranged so that his care is more convenient for the caregivers. Special foods may be necessary; a routine for all of the demanding physical care must be worked out. The boy's physical condition and emotional state are the central focus of the family. He has never had so much power. The friends of the parents rally around to help, but often it's hard to talk about anything other than the son's disability. It is an unnatural situation, one for which there aren't clear rules of behavior. The same is true for the young boy's friends. Some remain in contact, but many stay away because they don't know what to say or do, and are afraid of saying or doing the wrong thing. Siblings' relationships are also disrupted. They might choose to have fewer after-school or over-night guests than they did when the paraplegic was just a big brother.

Common Realities

Forms and prognoses of disabilities and chronic illnesses differ greatly. Some challenges such as blindness, deafness, and paraplegia are physically limiting but not life-threatening. Some chronic illnesses such as cancer, AIDS, and cystic fibrosis may take the individual's life. Other conditions, such as diabetes and most forms of hypertension, are controllable with medication, diet, and stress reduction. Illnesses that have been chronic for years can suddenly be cured by the discovery of a new drug or even occasionally by a religious or spiritual experience. But most illnesses don't follow these patterns; they must be managed through periods of remission and during times when the disease is active.

Despite differences in the forms and eventual outcomes of chronic illnesses and disabilities, they all result in common realities for those of us who have them. We all lose some kind of function; we are all in some way restricted. Freedom of choice and flexibility is reduced in our lives. To a greater or lesser degree, the illness or disability controls us and sets the boundaries for our thoughts, feelings, and actions. And we all suffer emotional pain.

This is where the challenge comes in. First, we are challenged to create our individual response to the uncertainty and limitations of our social and emotional lives. Second, and perhaps even more difficult, is the challenge to sustain our self-esteem in a society that sees us as different and somehow second-class. Third, we are challenged to make others comfortable with our limitations. In social relationships between disabled and nondisabled people, the disabled carry the burden of managing the situation so that others are not anxious or upset.

As we are challenged, each of us is forced to change. We may stretch or we may shrink, but we must change. We can choose to allow our lives to revolve increasingly around our physical condition. Or we can choose to commit ourselves to spiritual growth, refusing to let our physical condition limit the boundaries of our souls. We can choose to have spiritual health overcome physical illness or disablement.

Commitment to spiritual growth is not easy. Over and over we are tripped up by old habits, old ways of feeling and responding. There is no final fulfillment; we never reach some ultimate spiritual "goal." But in our struggle toward spiritual wellness we find little miracle after little miracle, and one day serenity may surprise us. We think, "Things are different. I am different. I am happy. I feel peace." The feeling may not stay with us for long; but once it has come, our reality has shifted in a deep and basic way. We have permanently changed. Our choice has taken hold.

For chronically ill and physically challenged people who choose this way, the question is, What are the obstacles we face if we choose our souls over our bodies? We clearly understand what our bodies struggle with, but what stands in the way of our spirit?

CHAPTER THREE

What's the Problem?

When you live with a chronic illness or a disability, "What's the problem?" may seem like a silly question. Physically, our lives are limited to one degree or another. We tend to think a lot about our condition and often need to plan our lives around it. In many cases, this is realistic. Yet many of us make our limits the focus of how we live, and we allow realistic limitations to spread unrealistically into areas of our lives where they don't belong.

A man with chronic heart problems becomes so focused on his situation that he limits his exercise and relationships so that he won't stress himself unnecessarily. Or perhaps he goes to the other extreme, spending hours walking, running, and playing tennis while avoiding a social life so that he won't be faced with tempting food and drink. An older woman who loses her sight can no longer tell where the food is on her plate. This very real limitation extends to, "I can't go out to eat because I can't see my food." This eventually leads to, "My life is so restricted, what's the use of it all?" A woman having chemotherapy loses her hair, hates how she looks in a wig, and stops socializing with her friends. A middle-aged male diabetic is impotent and avoids physical intimacy with his wife.

In this chapter we will discuss the emotional pain associated with physical limitations. In chapter 4 we will show how to cope with that pain and how to alleviate it.

Almost always, the way we behave in response to our illness or disability is based on pain—but the pain may be emotional, not physical. We who are in some way impaired share chronic, and sometimes overwhelming, emotional pain. We fear our condition will get worse and eventually kill us. At times we feel helpless, hopeless, trapped, even desperate. We may become depressed, grieving for the selves we once were. We may become enraged, shouting, "I hate it, I hate it, take it away." We may be ashamed and isolate ourselves, believing that we are worthless and that no one can understand. We may become exhausted from trying to cope. The intensity of emotional pain varies from person to person, and some of us are more troubled by one kind than another, but we all experience it.

It seems contradictory that emotional pain can contribute to our spiritual development. By itself, it would seem to destroy spirituality. In her pamphlet *Shame Faced,* Stephanie E. says that spirituality and shame cannot coexist, that we must release shame or its negative emotion can diminish or destroy our spirit. Others tell us that in confronting and struggling with emotional pain, our spirits are strengthened and expanded. Our emotional pain is both our curse and our blessing. But it's hard to look at it this way; it *feels* like a curse.

Identifying Our Emotional Pain

One of our first tasks in dealing with emotional pain is to identify it and place it in context. First, we will label the different kinds of pain and then discuss some useful ways to help turn them into a positive force in our lives.

Powerlessness

Both chronic illnesses and disabilities can be uncontrollable and unpredictable. A deaf man will not ever hear; a young woman with systemic lupus erythematosis (a disorder of the immune system) doesn't know what the course of her disease will be. So when we become ill or disabled, we feel a loss of control. Early in life we have learned that to be in control means to be safe—our very survival depends on it.

Now, perhaps suddenly, we can no longer control the most basic thing in our life—our body. Loss of control feels like powerlessness, which may lead to feelings of helplessness, hopelessness, rage, or even panic and despair. Our self-esteem seems to decrease in direct proportion to the increase in our sense of powerlessness. It is not unusual for a disabled or chronically ill person to feel hopeless about life and think, "What good is life if I can't be like other people?" or to despair, "How can I feel like life is worth anything at all when I have to depend so much on other people?" Many of us become anxious or panic-stricken. We feel as if we have absolutely no control of our lives and are worthless.

The less powerful we feel, the harder we try to maintain

control over both our internal and external worlds. We try to manipulate and control our thoughts, feelings, and behavior. As a consequence, we become excessively pre-occupied with ourselves. We use any tool possible to gain a feeling of control, even sometimes playing on others' guilt to manipulate them. We may hate ourselves for doing this, but we'll take whatever kind of power we can get.

Frequently, we don't give ourselves credit for the healthy gains in control that we do make.

In rehab, a stroke patient learns to take five steps without help. For a few moments she feels triumphant, then quickly says, "That's not so much. What does it really matter? I'll probably never be able to go up and down the stairs at home." A recently blinded adolescent confidently walks across the room she has memorized. Excited, she spins around and trips over a toy her young brother has left on the floor. She bursts into tears.

Powerlessness may seem like a total curse. What blessing could it possibly bestow? In chapter 4, we will find that acceptance of powerlessness is the basic first step on the journey toward spiritual wellness. What seems to be our most basic emotional pain—the pain on which all our other pain is built—can become our ticket to freedom.

Fear and Anxiety

Fear plays a huge part in the emotional pain of the chronically ill and disabled. We are afraid of many things, including the process of our illness, the pain, the increasing loss of control, the outcome, the possibility of dying.

Heart patients, cancer patients, and patients with nervous system or immune system disorders are all afraid of recurrences. No matter how well we feel at breakfast, by lunchtime we may have felt something or noticed something suspicious about the way our bodies felt or moved, and we are sucked into the obsessive fear of a recurrence. Add to this the fear many of us have of the medical establishment. Our fear may be based on mistrust that was due to past experiences or on a mature understanding that doctors are not gods and most medicine is not miraculous. We are afraid of our treatment and of side effects that can be painful and debilitating. We have financial concerns which, as bills and worries about insurance coverage mount, often become major fears.

We also have fears relating to our families and friends. We are afraid of how they see us, how they feel about us, and how our condition affects their lives. Many people with degenerative illnesses spend hours fearing for the future of their loved ones—afraid of depleting family financial resources during the course of their disease, afraid of whether a spouse can support and take care of children as the illness gets worse, afraid that friends will feel increasingly obligated to help.

Fear is a sneaky emotion. It creeps up and grabs us when we aren't looking. It nibbles at the edge of our mind as we are watching a glorious sunset following a thunderstorm, driving down the freeway, looking at the snow slowly falling outside the window, or enjoying a moment full of love and serenity at a Thanksgiving dinner. At times of normal activity, intense joy, or contentment, fear may whisper in our ear and the energy that was happiness may have to be used to put down fear, robbing our spirit.

Then there is anxiety, the way our mind protects us from fear. When we become too afraid of our fear, our mind often simply blanks it out with the buzzing of anxiety or panic. We can't function. The anxiety associated with fear can, in itself, become chronically disabling.

Yet fear can also bless us. We can recognize fear as a separate and manageable psychological response to emotional pain. We can learn that fear is only fear. This understanding is the key that allows us to choose how we are going to respond to powerlessness, isolation, anger, grief, or any of the other kinds of pain that we experience in our illness or disability. We can choose fear, or we can replace it with hope and faith.

Self-Pity

Chronically ill and physically challenged people regret their condition. It's a natural reaction. "This is a terrible thing that's happened to me!" is a cry that anyone might make under the circumstances. It is even to be expected that the next comment would be, "How awful for me to have to live this way." The problem arises when this natural regret slips into self-pity and becomes, "Poor me, poor me, poor me."

Those of us who feel the pain of self-pity don't see any way out of our situation. Our whole world increasingly revolves around ourselves, and we become almost completely self-absorbed.

"How can I possibly go on that backpacking trip? I'd have to live with a bunch of other people!" says Linda, who has a colostomy. "I couldn't possibly dress and undress with them around, and I might have to use communal toilets—how would I hide my colostomy bag? It's just totally selfish of you not to think of how terrible that would be for me. If you loved me, you'd think of my pain first."

Linda's response to her husband's suggestion of a hiking trip in the Sierras is typical of those of us who have let ourselves become obsessed with self-pity. We can see nothing in the world except our own pain. We try to manipulate others into making our pain a central part of their thinking process too. If that doesn't work, we rage at them or attempt to make them feel guilty in some other way. At first, those around us try to understand, and do things to appease us. But eventually they get tired of our incessant self-pity and turn away. Then we feel even sorrier for ourselves and the cycle continues. There is only one end to this path, and that is to add another emotional kind of pain to our already heavy load—the pain of isolation.

Isolation

The feeling of isolation is an emotional pain that can become overpowering. Whether we have a new illness or a long-term disability, we often feel alone and somehow outside the "normal" world. We may feel alone even among those who love and care for us. No one seems to understand our feelings. We are different, and there is no way to wipe away that difference.

When a man sits in a wheelchair, or a woman shakes with cerebral palsy, their difference is obvious. It is also apparent in the way they are treated by others. Often, when obviously disabled people are in a group, either an abundance of self-conscious attention is given them, or they are benignly ignored. This treatment, in itself, intensifies isolation and feelings of differentness.

People with conditions not obvious to an observer often feel isolated too. They feel helpless to explain themselves, or they expend emotional energy trying to pass as physically healthy.

A middle-aged woman recently diagnosed with lung cancer has lunch with a group of friends. When asked how things are in her life, she says, "Absolutely fine," and feels as alone as she has ever felt. An older man, athletic all of his life but now in an early stage of Parkinson's disease, avoids helping his hostess serve coffee because he can't trust himself to carry the cups. He excuses himself and goes into the bathroom, where he leans against the wall with feelings of despair and loneliness.

The antidote for isolation is involvement with others. A person might wonder why the chronically ill and disabled don't resolve their loneliness by reaching out. There are many reasons. We don't reach out because we don't want pity. We don't reach out because we don't want to have to explain. We don't reach out because we don't want to appear weak, as if we can't cope or keep a stiff upper lip. When we say we have lupus, heart disease, or cancer, we then become *identified* as having it and that makes it more real. We can't fool ourselves into pretending for even a little while that the condition isn't really there. Finally, and perhaps most devastating, we don't reach out because we are ashamed.

Feelings of shame and isolation are wound together in a knotted ball. We feel ashamed that we are different, that we aren't perfect, that perhaps somehow we are responsible for our condition. We feel ashamed of our physical weakness, or feel we are grotesque, or think of ourselves as a source of contamination. Our feelings of shame lead us to fears about how to present ourselves to others. Ultimately, shame leads to self-absorption, lowered self-esteem, and increased isolation.

But there is a potential blessing in the pain of isolation. First, we are forced to reach out to others to relieve it, and to join the human community everyone needs to become spiritually whole. Second, when we use the Twelve Steps to help ourselves work through the pain of isolation, we may trade isolation for aloneness. Aloneness can be a peaceful time in which to meet and understand our true selves—and to learn that we can survive.

Anger and Rage

People with chronic illness and disability experience anger and rage differently, depending on individual personality and upbringing.

When Marilyn describes her rage at her unrelenting, severe, disfiguring psoriasis (a chronic skin disease), she says, "Sure,

I'm really angry about it all, but if I think about my anger it feels more like despair or pleading. When I talk about being angry, there isn't much feeling in it. But if I think how the anger looks inside my head—it's just a flaming, rolling red mass."

This internal conflict reflects what many of us have learned about anger: We may have it, but we shouldn't express it. Some people, on the other hand, have no difficulty feeling and expressing their anger, and they rage at their condition. "God! When I think about it I could kill!" is not an unusual reaction.

Different aspects of our challenges bring out anger and rage. Some of us are angry because our bodies have betrayed us; others are angry because of a sense of powerlessness. Some of us are angry about the meaninglessness of our illness, some at the person or situation we blame for causing it. Some people's anger comes from feelings of jealousy and resentment or from a sense of being trapped. Many of us rage when we feel caught in the spiral of recurrence.

We may be angry at a lot of different things: God, nature, life, the world, medicines, doctors, treatments, hospitals. We get angry at family and friends for not understanding us, for not responding exactly as we want them to at a certain moment. We get angry when people make allowances for us, or when they don't. We may rage at our caregivers, alienating them or turning them into martyrs. We may displace our rage onto other things: our children's behavior, other drivers, or politicians. The world within our mind can be filled with free-floating rage.

We often project our anger on others, believing they are angry with us for something we did or didn't do. Anger can become a powerful tool and a way that we manipulate others. Our rage can take the form of self-destructive behaviors, such as drug abuse, suicide attempts, or reckless driving. Perhaps our anger is just too much to deal with, so we suppress it and become despondent or depressed.

The real power of rage and anger is that it has energy, lots and lots of energy. This energy will be useful if we turn it away from self-destruction and use its strength as an emotional basis for growth. We can transform the energy of anger into determination—determination to stretch our physical boundaries, and determination to expand our spiritual selves. Much as a rocket needs the massive thrust of flaming energy for blastoff, redirecting the energy of rage can propel us toward the heights of emotional wellness.

Blame and Ambiguity

Most of us certainly don't feel ambiguous about our illnesses or disabilities—we just don't want them. But we have them and somehow have to make sense of them. Before we can accept or adapt to anything in life, we have to make sense of it. We have to give it meaning. When we are struck with a chronic illness or become disabled, we feel a need to understand what it means. To do this, we must decide who or what is responsible for our condition. Here is where blame enters the picture. When something of little consequence happens to us, we can accept the responsibility for it easily. But when the event is very negative, we have all kinds of painful emotions and look for someone or something to blame. Our question becomes, "Whose fault is this?"

We often feel ambiguous about the answer. Do we blame fate, a doctor's misdiagnosis, faulty medical treatment, our mother's genes, or another person who caused the accident? Do we put the blame on an external source? Or do we internalize it, shaming ourselves for what we didn't do to prevent whatever it was that hurt us? Blaming others often turns into rage that generalizes into many areas of our lives; blaming ourselves often leads to self-hatred and depression.

No matter in which direction we point the finger of blame, there is no peace for us, so some people try a different approach. They sidestep the issue of fault by redefining the condition.

The mother whose adolescent son, now a quadriplegic, drove into a ditch while drunk, says, "He was driving home from a party at church and swerved to avoid a young couple walking their dog along the edge of the road."

She actually comes to believe that the accident occurred because of a self-sacrificing act on her son's part. The negative emotion is buried in a positive context, and she has peace without blame.

A woman who is diagnosed in her mid-thirties with multiple sclerosis says, "This must be God's way of telling me to reorganize the priorities in my life."

Now she no longer has to worry about whose fault her illness is. Whether or not we agree with this kind of mental gymnastics, it does help make sense of the situation, avoid ambiguity, and relieve the pain associated with blaming.

Blame and ambiguity are particularly hard for those of us with illnesses that go into remission and then recur. Every time we have a remission, we wonder what we, or someone else, did that caused it. When there's a recurrence, many of us think, "What did I do to make it worse? Should I change my diet, vitamins, exercise, or medication?" We try harder and harder to figure it out, putting more and more pressure on ourselves, wondering, "What's wrong with me that I can't manage this?"

New methods of stress reduction, mental imagery, and positive thinking add another dimension to the problem of self-blame. These are wonderful techniques that can be extremely beneficial in reducing strain on our already overtaxed systems, but they are not often going to cure us. A man with heart disease who spends time every day meditating and visualizing his heart as being strong and healthy can bring down his blood pressure, perhaps reduce his medication, feel much more serene, and live a happier life. However, this man will continue to be at an above-average risk of stroke or heart attack. This is not his fault. His efforts have helped control his disease. He is not to blame for the fact that he isn't cured.

As we consciously think through our responses of ambiguity and blame, we can begin to unravel the meaning of our illness or disability. This, in turn, helps expose the denial that keeps us stuck within our emotional pain. We learn to assign realistic responsibility, which helps us see our situation clearly. Our mind becomes unclouded by blaming, and our spirit becomes free of confusion.

Jealousy

Envy, resentment, and jealousy are emotional reactions that are very hard to separate from each other and very hard to eliminate. In our culture, many values and beliefs are deeply rooted in competition. To envy is to wish we had something that someone else has. To resent is to be angry and bitter because we don't have what someone else has. To be jealous is to have feelings of anger, sometimes hatred, toward the person who has what we want. Because so much emphasis is placed on perfection, none of us escapes feelings of jealousy, envy, and resentment from time to time. But when we are struck with a chronic illness or disability, these feelings can become a monumental influence in our lives.

We are resentful because we are different. We envy and are jealous of people whose lives are not impaired by illness and disability. We often resent people who move and speak easily and don't live with fear about the betrayal of their bodies. We may envy what we see as the freedom of their lives.

A young girl in a wheelchair watches from her front porch as her neighborhood friends go off to the swimming pool. She is jealous of the other girls. She is concentrating on things that they can do that she cannot. Instead of appreciating her own skill on the flute, she envies her friends. Her emotional energy is used for jealousy, and she forgets what a fantastic time she and those same girls had yesterday playing Trivial Pursuit.

Jealousy keeps this girl focused on the impossible; she forgets her own potential. Yet those of us who are cursed with jealousy can also experience its gift. When we use the Twelve Steps and commit ourselves to release our jealousy, we can learn to stop comparing ourselves with others. We learn to value ourselves as incredibly wonderful, unique people, important and acceptable just as we are.

Grief

It is necessary and normal for us to experience grief with the onset of a disability or chronic illness. "Necessary and normal" doesn't lessen the pain; it simply says that we are going to grieve.

The woman who takes her stroke "like a brick" is hiding her grief. Perhaps she is trying to take care of herself, or maybe to take care of those around her—but her attitude will limit her ability to truly come to peace with her condition.

After years spent working with terminally ill patients, Dr. Elisabeth Kübler-Ross described the grief process associated with death. Her work *On Death and Dying* is still considered a classic in the field. Now scholars teach us that the grief process is associated with all loss, whether it is moving from one home to another, getting married or divorced, or becoming disabled or chronically ill.

All change involves loss, even happy change. When

we get married, we are happy to begin a new life with a beloved person; at the same time we grieve for lost parts of our single life. If we have a second child, we may grieve the loss of the little family we had until that time. When we are disabled or develop a chronic illness, we will grieve for the person that we were, the life that we had been living, our changed relationships, or our lost future.

Some griefs are small, some are large, some almost overwhelm us—but whatever the degree, the process is the same. There are three phases of grief. The first stage is denial, which involves shock, numbness, and disbelief.

Seventeen-year-old Jake has been in a hospital for three weeks. He is out of intensive care and recovering, but a diving accident has left him a quadriplegic. Jake simply cannot believe that he will never walk again. He feels numb, not comprehending his situation. He tells friends, "The doctors say this is permanent, but they don't know me!" His mother can't believe it either: "I just don't seem able to feel anything."

People with illnesses or disabilities that aren't obvious often get stuck in this phase as they continually try to pass as "normal." The denial associated with being "normal" keeps them from moving toward acceptance of their condition.

The second phase of grief is one of intense emotional pain. Extreme mood swings, overwhelming sadness, raging grief, depression, lethargy, hyperactivity, regression to childlike helplessness, despair, guilt, and bargaining with doctors or God—all these are emotions and behaviors that can possess us.

This second phase also includes anger. We may be angry at everyone and everything. We may lash out toward others or turn anger inward on ourselves. The greater the loss, the less prepared for it we are, the more limited our options, the longer anger may continue. The danger is that we will get stuck in it.

While grief is normal, its course is not predictable. We jump from phase to phase and back again. The important thing is that grief must be dealt with slowly, over a long period of time. There will be many regressions, but we must keep actively aware of the process. Some people come to a point in their cycle of grief where they just stop—they get stuck and grief becomes chronic. They continue to promise God that they will never smoke again if He will remove their lung cancer. They stay deeply depressed, refusing to do things to relieve their depression. Soon, depression becomes a way to manipulate those around them. They refuse to care for their bodies, insisting that a caregiver feed and dress them. They wallow in guilt and rage at the world.

Ultimately, most people with a stable disability or unremitting disease move beyond these first phases of grief. On the other hand, people with illnesses that have periods of remission and recurrence can easily get stuck. Every time their illness retreats, hope springs up, and hope begets denial. Then when, inevitably, illness recurs, the second phase of grief starts all over again. These people may have a very hard time moving on to the final stage of the process.

In the third phase of grief we learn to let go of the past

and to accept ourselves as we are. We learn to live with our situation and to look forward again. Even people with terminal illness tell us that they can find acceptance, peace, and a sense of the future. Their future may be measured in days or even hours, but their eyes and emotions are in the present. They look forward to seeing friends and loved ones, perhaps indulging in their favorite food or watching birds on a feeder. "Maybe this afternoon or tomorrow, the narcissus will bloom," they tell themselves. Many of them envision an afterlife reflecting their religious beliefs, and from this they gain hope.

The blessing of grief is in its process. We are thrown into grieving; we feel its pain and agony; yet we finally come to acceptance. To go through the grieving process gives us a deeply rooted faith that everything passes, that there is some way to deal with whatever we must deal with, and that we will come out into the light. Somehow, grief cleanses us; we are left ready to rebuild.

Exhaustion

Many of us with chronic illness or disability also suffer from chronic exhaustion. We can be overwhelmed by the physical barriers we face. Add to this the energy sapped by the emotional pain and negative feelings we live with, and it is no wonder we are tired.

The amount of sheer energy used by a stroke victim as she struggles with her walker to the bathroom; the sheer energy used by a paraplegic as he lowers himself from his van, wheels his chair across a sidewalk, and maneuvers to open a plate-

glass door; the sheer energy used by a woman with Parkinson's
as she negotiates the stairs in her apartment house—it all re-
sults in exhaustion, and it is their way of life.

It's hard to see how exhaustion can bless us. Like severe
depression, it leaves us drained and passionless. But when
we feel empty and at the end of our rope, there is, for
most of us, an instinctive urge toward survival. Within
our deepest core we look for a way to connect with living.
We may be physically and emotionally tired, but spiritually we find strength to help ourselves.

Breaking Out of the Pain Cycle

We've been talking about the emotional pain that unites
chronically ill and disabled people. Unfortunately, many
of our cultural beliefs and religions don't help relieve the
pain. As young children, we may have learned that we
will get what we deserve in life. For chronically ill or disabled people, this translates into, "I must be pretty bad to
have had this happen to me," a thought that creates guilt
and lowered self-esteem. We may have been taught that
suffering ennobles a person. You may say, "I have to be a
good sport about this, pretend that everything's great,
even though I hate it with all my heart." We reject our
grief and crush its process. We may have been taught that
everything that happens, happens for a purpose. Trans-
lation: "If this has happened to me, there must be a reason. I've got to figure out what it is." Such an idea can
mean months, perhaps years, of fruitless struggle to find
meaning in a purposeless, life-diminishing accident.

It would be wrong to say that chronically ill and disabled people are constantly experiencing, or being overwhelmed by, emotional pain. But it is a significant and crippling part of our lives. For many of us, the unresolved anger, grief, and feelings of powerlessness keep our spiritual development stuck, cycling round and round rather than taking a straight path toward growth. In doing this, we increase the negative effects of our illness and the extent of our disability.

To break out of the cycle, we can work through our pain and replace it with determination, satisfaction, contentment, happiness, joy, and serenity. Although each of us brings a unique personality to this task, we can all reexamine our lives and values. We can fight denial and accept the unacceptable. We can decide that our lives are worth living, even with the illness or disability that we suffer, and that we can find spiritual meaning.

The Twelve Step program gives us a map for our spiritual growth. The Steps were built on the premise that alcoholism is a spiritual illness as well as a chronic, degenerative physical process. Those of us who suffer chronic illness or disability have a spiritual illness too. Our spiritual illness has grown out of emotional pain, which keeps us focused on our physical condition and stunts our spiritual growth. The Twelve Steps offer us a new way to live. They provide a way to turn the threat of our illness or disability into a challenge toward living a full life. By making them the pattern for our lives, we will achieve a spiritual wellness that becomes more important than our physical condition. We will find serenity and joy.

CHAPTER FOUR

The Twelve Step Journey

The emotional pain connected to our physical condition has a destructive effect on our spirituality. It keeps us cycling around our illness or disability and we can't grow in a more productive way. The Twelve Step program provides a way of life that relieves the emotional pain we live with and offers a design for reaching spiritual health.

The Twelve Step journey is to be taken one day at a time and at a pace that is comfortable. We accept the First Step and make it a part of our lives—followed by the Second, Third, Fourth, and so on, through the entire program. As we work a Step, we may have new insights about an earlier one, so we go back and think some more, making changes or additions to what we had done before. The objective is to continually deepen our understanding and to translate this into the way we live our lives.

The Steps are not a test—speed, competitiveness, correctness, and perfection aren't relevant. The goal is our individual spiritual wellness. We reach this goal by feeding our spirit as we move from Step to Step. We learn to accept ourselves and our lives, release our pain, and deepen our spiritual awareness. Almost no one experiences a spiritual awakening as a single inspirational event. Instead, we have one small awakening after another, and they add up. This new philosophy, this new way of life, is not easily gained.

It takes great patience, effort, and tolerance to get through the times when we slip back into old ways. Slips are to be expected; old habits will fight hard to stay with us.

But the Twelve Steps will help us. They suggest humility; a willingness to face facts; a freedom from false pride, grandiosity, and arrogance. They suggest honesty, freedom from self-deception, sincerity in our desire to eliminate our pain, and a willingness to admit that we have been following an unhealthy path. They suggest faith—a belief in a Power greater than our own individual will from which we can draw strength. They suggest courage, the fortitude to endure the things we cannot change, and the appreciation of the ways we can change. Finally, they suggest service—reaching out to others who need and want the same kind of help that we have needed and wanted. When we change our old ways of being, and carefully and consciously live as the Twelve Steps instruct, our spirituality will be slowly enriched, and we will become more than we have ever been.

Following are the Twelve Steps of AA, adapted for our condition of chronic illness or disability. At the end of each Step there are exercises to use as the Step is practiced. Because of differing personalities, some people will prefer the written exercise, some the imagery, some will use both, and others will make up a unique exercise to fit their own needs. It doesn't matter. Just do it.

The written exercises will be most helpful if you answer in as much detail as possible. Take plenty of time—hours, days, even months. There are no "correct" answers, and speed is not important. We are working toward long-term change, and it is the thoughtfulness and depth of response that matter.

The imagery exercises are designed to help you incorporate each Step into your life. They are not magic; but if practiced repeatedly and sincerely, they are one of the most powerful tools we have to achieve spiritual growth. Freed from your control, your subconscious mind will tell you what you already know but cannot reach. Everyone images differently—there is no "right" way. Some people see pictures in their minds; some simply have sensations or feelings that represent the contents of the image. However it works for you, accept it.

Powerless Yet Powerful

Step One: We admitted we were powerless over our chronic illness or disability—that our lives had become unmanageable.*

Step One asks us to admit that our chronic illness or disability causes us emotional pain, that we are powerless over this pain, that we cannot control it, move away from it, or manage it. To most of us, this is an appalling idea. We have struggled hard with our condition and don't want to admit our powerlessness over the emotional pain it causes us. We spend our energy denying, pretending

---

* The Twelve Steps for Chronically Ill or Disabled People quoted in these chapters are an adaptation of the Twelve Steps of Alcoholics Anonymous. This adaptation was done with the permission of Alcoholics Anonymous World Services. The original Twelve Steps of Alcoholics Anonymous appear in appendix A. See editor's note on copyright page.

that our physical condition is what matters, ignoring the fact that our emotional pain is a problem in itself.

Sarah, a thirty-six-year-old wife and mother of two children, has systemic lupus erythematosis. "I work so hard at managing it. I use healing imagery, watch my diet like a hawk, do everything the doctors suggest, exercise, and almost kill myself trying to use positive thinking. I just can't believe that I don't have control over this disease! If I believed that, it would be like giving up, and giving up means dying."

Sarah defines her fears and anxieties as emotions "not to give in to" because then she might "give up" and die.

Brad, fifty, is quite crippled. When he was thirty-five he was diagnosed with multiple sclerosis and has struggled to maintain all the physical function he could. Many, many times he yearned to give up, to stop working so hard for so little, trying to hold back the onslaught of complete dysfunction. "But," he says, "if I hadn't done my damnedest to stay in control over this thing, I might be completely helpless by now."

Brad denies that emotional pain plays any part in his struggle.

Ella has had cerebral palsy since birth. Every day for forty-two years she has fought to keep herself in control—to be as much like other women as she could. "Control, manage, control, manage—those two words hold the story of my life. They're what I know best in the world."

Ella can't describe serenity.

What these valiant people say is true. They take responsibility for themselves, they work at controlling their lives, they constantly try to manage, but while they control and manage, they deny the importance of their emotional pain.

For those of us who live with physical illness or disability, it is particularly difficult to accept the idea of personal powerlessness. We are accustomed to working hard to deal with a physical condition that has been handed to us by fate. Most of us take full, active responsibility for our lives. We look strong, we cope, but we can't fool our psyche; our emotional pain does not go away. Instead, it remains unmanageable. It stays with us despite our best efforts and for just one reason: We continue to fight, deny, and attempt to overcome our powerlessness. We keep trying to manage the unmanageable while the feelings of helplessness, hopelessness, rage, panic, despair, fear, anxiety, jealousy, and grief continue.

The First Step is the foundation of the Twelve Step program. It is not meant as a Step in which we judge ourselves. It is an opportunity to objectively observe our behavior and admit that we cannot continue alone, that we need help. Admitting this need for help is a way of surrendering, and this breaks through our denial and lets us be honest with ourselves.

To Surrender Is to Win

For our logical mind, surrender as victory may be a hard concept to understand. Perhaps it will help to look at the postures of t'ai chi, the ancient Chinese ritual dance of life.

If we study t'ai chi, we find that the posture for Strength is to stand erect, arms extended straight out to the side from the shoulders, palms turned upward, legs straight, and feet planted firmly on the ground. The entire body is held in firm control, pressing upward as if to support an immense load of weight, fully engaged with external pressure. This strong pose begins the dance, which then flows into the Chinese posture of Power.

In Power, the legs remain straight, feet solidly grounded, but the arms and shoulders curve in. The head drops to the chest, and the entire upper body is rounded, pulled in, curved down toward the abdomen. To us in the Western world this looks like a pose of abject surrender; but to the Chinese it represents gathering in, protecting the life energy within the very center of the body. There is disengagement with external stress, and the body presents a form that the pressures of the world can pour over, slide down, and flow away from. Strength uses up energy, while Power conserves and increases it.

The First Step asks us to stop carrying the weight of our whole world. Instead, it suggests we give up our struggles to manage, gather in our energy, bend down, and hold it within ourselves.

As we work the First Step, we are asked to put aside the pride that has taken so much of our energy. We are asked to become humble. Humility does not mean giving up our selfhood, nor does it mean to bow down in a servile manner. Humility is about equality and place. People have less power than nature and are certainly humbled before it. But without human beings, nature is incomplete. To become humble is to accept our place in the overall scheme of life, without arrogance or grandiosity. Everyone and everything is important and is equally necessary in creating and maintaining the whole.

The First Step also asks that we admit our obsessive need to control and manage. It asks that we accept our powerlessness over our emotional pain. It tells us that our spiritual journey to serenity begins with surrender. In the past, the satisfaction we experienced when we had everything under control might have been called a kind of serenity. But that serenity could be instantly threatened— at any moment we could lose control. The serenity we experience when we give up our attempts to maintain everlasting control, when we surrender to our powerlessness, can never be threatened—we have no control to lose.

To Surrender Is Not to Quit

"Surrender" is a frightening word to many of us. We surrender in wartime to our enemies. We surrender something when we give it up to someone else. We surrender when we quit. As very young children we may have been taught that good guys win and losers surrender—so, by the definition we understand, those who surrender are quitters and losers. We sometimes hear that we surrender in love, but even then surrendering has an overtone of weakness.

Sarah believes that if she surrenders, she will die. Brad thinks surrender would mean total helplessness, and Ella has had a life so full of holding on to control that the concept of surrender is as foreign to her as the world of science fiction.

But if we think about it, there are wonderful aspects to surrender. If we surrender to our sense of powerlessness, we have a potential for getting real help and nurturing.

If Sarah surrenders the outcome of her condition, she can be more realistic in expending her limited energy and ask those who love her to support her in ways that can make her life less frantic and more meaningful. Brad can gain relief from putting down the impossible burden that he has tried to carry alone. He can feel closer to his wife and accept her help. Finally, Ella can find relief from the pressure of trying to belong that has plagued and narrowed her life. In surrender she can learn how serenity feels.

Surrender does not mean giving up responsibility for our actions or our emotional pain. It does mean understanding and accepting the fact that we cannot control the outcome of our condition, that we are powerless over the pain it brings us. When we acknowledge this, our healing begins. The emotional energy that has been bound in pain is released, and we can use it for intimacy, love, and creativity. In our surrender to powerlessness, we find energy for the powerful emotions that can lead us to spiritual health.

Step One: Written Exercise

1. When you look back on your life, how important has control been to you?

2. Does the concept of powerlessness or surrender frighten you? Why?

3. What difficulties are you having in (a) recognizing your powerlessness over the emotional pain attached to your illness or disability, and (b) recognizing that your life has become unmanageable?

4. How is your emotional pain affecting your current life?

5. How do you define *humility*? What do you believe are its positives and negatives?

6. How do you define *surrender*? What do you believe are its positives and negatives?

7. If you were relieved of your emotional pain, how would your life change?

Step One: Imagery Exercise

Close your eyes and allow an image of yourself to come into your mind. Picture yourself walking in the woods. You are carrying a heavy backpack that strains at the seams. Try to imagine this backpack in detail—its color, size, how it fits on your back. Does it have a frame? Or is it supported by your neck and shoulders alone? If you have never carried a pack, just imagine what it looks like and how it feels to carry its weight.

Imagine that this pack carries everything you need to control all of the pain, all of the power you try to maintain, and all of the managing skills that you've worked so hard for. As you keep walking through the woods, you stumble every now and then over rocks or exposed roots in the path. You have to keep your eyes down—your head pulls forward to support the weight on your back. Feel the strain in your neck and shoulders. Look at the path under your feet. You can't look upward, or even very far forward, because that would throw you off balance and you might fall.

Imagine that the path ends at the edge of a meadow. With your peripheral vision you barely see long green grass, bending in the light breeze. Blue forget-me-nots and white daisies are in bloom. Feel yourself standing on the edge of this meadow, yearning to run free or to lie down in the fragrant grass and rest with the sun pouring its energy into you. But to do this, you must first put down your pack. You can neither run nor rest while carrying this load.

Now do it. Swing the pack off of your shoulders and let it drop. Hear the crunching sound it makes as it hits the ground. Take a moment to enjoy the feeling of lightness and relief. Straighten up, raise your head, just stand there, and savor the release. Begin to move away from the pack; it lies there at the edge of the meadow and soon you can't see it anymore. Allow yourself to feel the freedom. It's all right, you don't have to feel guilty or afraid, just relish the lightness. You've left your need to control and to manage in that pack. Now you are powerless and free, powerless and full of a feeling of confidence, comfort, and serenity.

Just for now, don't think about what happens to your power, who gets it, or where it goes. As a controller, you are always straining to meet the future before it comes, but now you must learn to take one step at a time. Simply feel the freedom that comes with putting down your load. PERIOD. Feel the freedom and get used to it—it's the First Step.

Open your eyes and resume your life. During the day, stop for a moment now and then. Remember the feeling of freedom you had when you put down the pack and admitted you were powerless by dropping all your efforts at control.

Finding Our Own Power Source

Step Two: Came to believe that a Power greater than ourselves could restore us to sanity.

The Twelve Step program first requires that we admit our powerlessness and change our controlling, managing, manipulative behaviors. Then it asks that we accept the unconditional existence of a spiritual force, a Power greater than ourselves, which we are willing to believe can heal our emotional pain. The First Step suggests the change we need to make in our way of thinking; the Second Step lays the spiritual basis for the program.

"Came to believe that a Power greater than ourselves . . ."
This phrase often causes confusion, misunderstanding, and outright rejection of the Twelve Step program. Many, many people hear it and say, "I'm not a religious person; I just cannot believe in God." They don't understand that neither God nor religion is the issue. What is at issue is accepting the existence of some Power outside of ourselves that offers spiritual resources to help us.

Many of us who struggle with chronic illness or disability have come to believe in self-sufficiency. As a consequence, we become isolated in many ways. Our self-sufficiency has created barriers between both ourselves and other people and ourselves and a Higher Power. Even for those of us who believe in a traditional God, it may be hard to place Him in our lives. He certainly hasn't taken away our condition or made clear why we must suffer. Some of us are agnostics, some atheists. Many of us have never taken the time or made the effort to develop our own spiritual philosophy. Seriously considering what we believe about life, about living, and about how the universe operates is hard work and takes time. Other things are more pressing. The living of life takes precedence over the contemplation of it.

Also, we tend to confuse religion with spirituality. We believe that if we think about "spiritual" things, then we must somehow tie them to a "religious" belief. When we try to understand the meaning of "Came to believe that a Power greater than ourselves . . . ," the first thing we need to do is to separate religion and spirituality. The Twelve Steps is a spiritual program, not a religious one. When we talk about spirituality, we are talking about the spirit of life. Spirituality is an enigma that we cannot see, or touch, or measure. It is made up of the forces that make life happen. For religious people, this life force may be God. For people who do not have traditional religious beliefs, it will be something else.

Developing Our Spirituality

Neither religious nor scientific thinkers can agree about what spirituality is or where it is located. Most of us are not philosophers; we can't argue the fine points of science and spiritual or religious doctrine. But we can think through a spiritual philosophy for ourselves. While our personal philosophy may change and deepen over time, the important thing for us to do now is to begin. That is what the Second Step asks of us.

Our willingness to surrender and believe in the process of the Twelve Steps helps us let go of our self-will. When this happens, a block is removed and our subconscious becomes much more available to us. It may give us messages in dreams and odd, fleeting thoughts. Strange coincidences tend to occur. We may recognize signs of a presence of which we have been totally unaware. Slowly the idea of a "Power greater than ourselves" becomes easier to grasp and more acceptable. As we stop trying to single-handedly manage our condition and the emotional pain that comes with it, we begin to think that perhaps some kinds of spiritual resources might help us.

There are no rules for the form our individual Higher Power will take. It can be whomever or whatever we choose. Some choose God as they understand Him or Her. Some choose an image in their mind. Some choose human love, nature, or the universe. Some choose the Twelve Step program itself. Higher Powers, spiritual resources, are whatever give us strength, hope, and serenity and enhance our humanity. The form simply isn't important. All that matters is the belief that the Power exists and is greater than we are. If we allow the belief to happen, our own individual Power will come to us.

Rhoda has kidney disease. Her life is limited by dialysis and the other protocols that go with her condition. She is Jewish, but left the practice of Judaism several years before, when she married a man who has no professed religious belief. Rhoda's Higher Power is an oak tree. "I know that sounds really silly, but when I look at a tree, particularly an oak tree, I know that there is something that controls our universe. When I call on my Higher Power, I also have some stirrings of old stuff from back in the days when I was practicing Judaism. But I'm not ready to deal with that now, and that wonderful oak tree does the job."

Judy, who has had uterine cancer, says, "After years and years of thinking I had no religious belief left from my childhood, I've found that my Higher Power is God—and He's the God that I knew from Sunday school. I feel as though I've come home."

Dan has been an atheist all of his life, just like his father. Also, just like his father, he has severe heart disease. Dan sees the Twelve Step program as his Higher Power. "It isn't the people in the program that I think of as my Higher Power, although they're a terrific support. It's the way the program is a representation of how all of us struggle, of our combined spiritual strength, and of our caring about each other—that's what helps me. There's a lot to this program. It can fit anyone. As they say, you can take what you want and leave the rest."

Meg was raised in a strict Catholic home. It has been fifteen years since she was blinded by a freak accident in her mid-

twenties. "I had a really hard time with this whole Higher Power idea. The God I had always known was a strict God, with rules and regulations that wouldn't quit. He was also vengeful. I could never make a mistake or He might send me to hell. I never felt that I could ask Him for anything, because there was no way I was good enough to deserve His help or consideration. So when I began to think about a Power greater than myself, I went back and reinvented God. It was terribly hard and took a long time. But I've done it! My God is an all-loving Father. I asked myself how it would feel to have a father that just loved me, the way I want to be loved, no matter what I did. And you can't imagine the peace and freedom I feel now."

Jane, a woman in her mid-sixties, is quite disabled by rheumatoid arthritis. She found her Higher Power by asking it to appear in her imagination—and it did. "For me, it's a huge white light. It is made up of all of the energy from all living things, and that includes inanimate objects, like rocks. They live, just in a different way. Anyhow, all of this energy is combined in a huge pool and it's there for the asking, for anyone. The wonder of it is that not only do we use it when we need to, but our very being puts more energy back into that pool so it can never run out."

". . . could restore us to sanity."
Is the Second Step calling us insane? Is it saying that our unhealthy attitudes and behavior, our emotional pain, is a kind of insanity? That's what the Step implies, and perhaps it's right. If we were completely rational observers,

objectively evaluating someone who thinks, feels, and acts as we do, many of those thoughts, emotions, and actions would seem irrational. This Step tells us that a Power greater than ourselves can help us release our irrationality and lead us to spiritual fulfillment.

There seem to be five major factors involved in spiritual fulfillment: spiritual strength, humility, understanding, emotional stability, and peace of mind. Let's take a closer look at each of them.

Spiritual strength develops from our recognition of a Higher Power and our faith in its healing. Spiritual strength also comes from thinking through a personal spiritual philosophy.

We find humility when we follow the Twelve Step program, give up our obsession with control and management, and truly accept our equality as human beings.

Understanding comes when we break through denial and self-absorption and realize that others struggle as we do.

Giving up our focus on our condition, and allowing ourselves to accept the love, care, and support of our Higher Power, can bring us emotional stability.

Surrendering to powerlessness over our condition and emotional pain, together with faith in the healing potential of our Higher Power, can give us peace of mind.

Perhaps when we think of spiritual fulfillment, it is more useful to think of spiritual *evolution*. To evolve means to change, unfold, become more complex, to be more than we have been in the past. It means to develop against the forces of habit and inertia, to extend ourselves beyond wherever we think we are able to go. It means to choose the force within us that pushes us toward the difficult path of growth and to transcend our chronic illness or disability and emotional pain.

As our Higher Power becomes more a part of our lives, we become more spiritually fulfilled. We come to accept, respect, and love ourselves just as we are, without qualification.

Now working the Twelve Steps, Meg says, "I don't really understand much of the philosophical talk, but what I do know is that I feel better than I have since I can remember. I'm not so angry, not so scared, and having a Higher Power seems to help me feel more in place."

Looking at reality, admitting our powerlessness over the situation, and being supported by a loving, caring Power greater than ourselves can remove our emotional pain. Rhoda's oak tree, Meg or Judy's God, Dan's Twelve Steps, or Jane's white light—any of these very individual Higher Powers will relieve us. The form doesn't matter, as long as it is ours, and as long as we believe in it.

Step Two is often referred to as the "Hope Step." It tells us that there is help available. There is a way out, a way so easy and yet so difficult. All we need to do is let go of our need to control our condition and the emotional pain that goes with it, and accept that there are spiritual resources greater than ourselves and ask them to help. We no longer need to struggle alone.

Step Two: Written Exercise

1. What does the statement "The Twelve Steps have a spiritual foundation" mean to you?

2. What differences do you see between religion and spirituality?

3. What fears or other roadblocks stand between you and your acceptance of a Higher Power?

4. If you decide to accept the existence of a Power greater than yourself, how do you think your life will change? Be specific.

5. Describe how self-will and self-absorption can block your acceptance of a Higher Power.

6. How does your childhood experience of religion and spirituality influence the way you believe today? How does it help you? How does this experience get in your way?

Step Two: Imagery Exercise

Close your eyes and imagine yourself alone somewhere—a neutral place, not wonderful and not frightening. Very carefully look at yourself. Take time to see your illness or disability exactly as it is and feel the emotional pain that goes with it. The pain may be a mishmash of nonspecific feelings, or it may be made up of very clear, negative, or frightening emotions. Just see yourself as you truly are and let the feelings wash over you.

Ask your Higher Power to join you. Look at Him or Her or It—whatever it is for you—and experience how you feel when it is with you, when you can see it or sense its presence.

Ask this Higher Power to help your painful feelings go away. Wait, be still, and see what happens. Perhaps you will feel relief, freedom, or gratitude; or maybe you will feel very little change. Whatever happens is all right—this exercise works differently for different people. Your Higher Power is yours alone and will help you in its own special way.

Open your eyes. You can repeat this exercise daily, maybe even several times a day. Allow time, and you will experience a change in your feelings and a lessening of your emotional pain.

CHAPTER FIVE

Gaining Strength through New Beliefs

As we work through the first two Steps, we begin to develop a personal philosophy—we make a commitment to connect with our own spiritual force. In Step Three, our commitment is tested because we must make an active decision to turn our will and lives over to this nebulous force outside of ourselves. For many of us, this is even more difficult than the first Steps. It calls for active surrender; and as chronically ill or disabled people, we are accustomed to trusting our own will, not surrendering to the will of others. When we are struggling with this idea, it helps to remember that we haven't done such a good job of managing up to this point; painful feelings and destructive emotions still make up a good part of our lives.

Power at Our Fingertips

Step Three: Made a decision to turn our will and our lives over to the care of the God of our understanding.

In the first three Steps we lay the groundwork for our entire recovery program; Steps Four through Twelve build on this foundation. For this reason, it is crucial that we feel comfortable with the first three Steps, that we feel truly able to carry out all that they ask. Take your time and review as much as necessary. There is no hurry. What is important is that we understand the ideas and accept the concepts.

"Made a decision to turn our will and our lives over . . ."
To "make a decision" is clear-cut and easy to understand. But what about "to turn over"? Just what does this mean? For some people working the Third Step, it means exactly what it says—to give away, to no longer have control over, to put whatever it is in the hands of someone or something else.

Meg believes that from the time she "turned it over," God took control of her life. She came to believe that He has a purpose for whatever happens to her and is always with her. God is Meg's active partner in every facet of her life. She truly believes "Thy will be done."

For Jane, "turning it over" is a more abstract concept. She believes that "to turn over" means to ask for support from her spiritual force, her White Light. It also means to present the Light with her concerns and to live by the ideals she believes it represents. Meg's life is guided by God's words from the Bible, while Jane has worked out a personal philosophy that includes her White Light. Their relationships with their Higher Powers are different, but both women are equally dedicated to the process. They may have different belief systems, but their underlying faith is the same. They each have faith that they are no longer operating alone—they have asked someone or something else to be the overlying power and influence in their lives.

The Third Step asks for "our will and our lives." This can be a frightening idea, since there would be nothing of us left without "our will and our lives." In a way this is true. Making a decision to turn over "our will and our lives" means that we no longer have sole control over ourselves. We now accept a spiritual force that we have committed to follow. But this does not mean that we give up and become passive.

On the contrary, most of us find that when we decide to turn "our will and our lives" over to a Power greater than ourselves, we are freed to become more active than we have ever been. Lots of emotional energy previously used to manage and control is now free. We can take realistic responsibility for our choices, our actions, our feelings, and the principles and values by which we live. We give up our willfulness as we search for beliefs and behaviors that reflect the will of our Higher Power. We work at our lives in a way that represents the ideals of God, or Light, or the Twelve Step program, or whatever spiritual resources help us. We surrender the outcome but retain responsibility in our lives. A saying very appropriate for the Third Step is "When you're out in a boat and a storm comes up, pray to God, and row as hard as you can toward shore."

At first, turning over "our will and lives" may be confusing and difficult to do. We may have a hard time seeing how all of this relates to our condition. Do we stop being actively involved in our own care? Of course not. We may become even more active in our role with doctors, therapists, and treatment, and more creative in the management of our disabilities. But our activity is different because, as we become deeply involved with our Higher Power, the emotional pain that has stood in our way begins to decrease.

Dan talks about how his relationship with his doctor has changed since he began to work the Twelve Steps. "In the beginning," he says, "I was so angry, just full of rage, and I didn't trust anybody—least of all the guy that was making me face up to my problem. Then as I got involved with the Twelve Steps, I got less angry and my defensiveness went away. I felt much more confident with my doc, and I could get my point across without the whole scene falling apart. When things got better and we began to have decent conversations, he thought they were just between us. If only he knew, I had the whole blasted Program with me every time."

". . . to the care . . ."

The Third Step tells us that we should turn over our will and our lives to the "care" of the God of our understanding, and "care" is a wonderful word. It means to be guided, inspired, supported, helped, and relieved of our emotional pain. To be cared for means to be unquestioningly and unequivocally nurtured.

When we are disabled or become seriously ill, the deepest and most immediate feeling we have is screaming, raging emotional pain. The small child who lives at our very core cries out to be taken care of, but no one hears. We try not to listen, and there is no comfort for that terrified little person. Yet miraculously, when we take the Third Step, the child begins to be comforted—our Higher Power hears and provides care. This becomes an unceasing process. Whether it is the small child within us who needs comforting, or the adult who needs help and support, the caring is always there.

". . . of the God of our understanding."
To whom or what do we turn over our "will and our lives"? Step Two gives us an idea or an image of our personal Higher Power. In Step Three, we begin to deepen that relationship. As we work to "turn our will and our lives over" to the God of our understanding, we need to ask for direction. We need to discover by what values and principles we should live. We need to turn to our Higher Power for support, to have its caring begin to remove our pain. We can learn to talk with our Higher Power and, over time, this becomes less a self-conscious act and more a natural part of life. When we have questions about a decision or a course of action, we ask for direction. When we need help or support, we ask. When we need to be relieved of pain, we ask. We learn to ask and then to be still and wait for the response. If we are still, if we are patient, if we believe, the response will come. There are sayings that can help us keep the faith:

- Turn it over to the Program.
- Release it to the Light.

- Let go, let God.
- One day at a time.

When we finish the first three Steps, we have laid the foundation for the rest of our Twelve Step work. It's a turning point. Here are three short studies of how this first part of the program has worked for three very different people: Meg, Jane, and Dan.

Meg's Story

The car accident that blinded Meg at age twenty-six also left her depressed.

"I couldn't, or wouldn't, even try to do all the retraining and therapy that is provided for blind people. I'd had three drinks that night and was convinced that the whole thing was my own fault. I was ashamed. I felt like I was no good to anyone, like my whole life was over. Actually, I wanted to die—don't know why I didn't. One of my therapists talked to me about religion, getting help from God, but the only God I understood would have blamed me just the way I blamed myself—so that idea was worse than useless."

After two years, Meg's depression lifted enough so that she could live alone, keep a job, and take care of herself, but she remained isolated, living a much more limited life than her blindness required. She was also crippled by anxiety.

"Then a woman at work suggested that I go with her to Al-Anon. She was kind. She said that if she could learn to live

with an alcoholic husband, I should be able to learn to live with my blindness. And at Al-Anon this tremendous thing happened. I got the chance to create my own Higher Power. It was okay to make up whatever kind of Power greater than myself I wanted to. So I made up my own God. I made Him to be just what I wanted—the perfect, loving Father. I turned myself over to Him, and He's involved in my whole life. All I have to do is say 'help,' and He's there. All my fear and anxiety and depression are gone. I didn't think you could be blind, normal, and happy, but I am."

Jane's Story

Jane, who is disabled with rheumatoid arthritis, tells how the program worked for her.

"I've had this disease most of my adult life—sometimes it's worse, sometimes it goes into remission, but the trend is always down, and it always will be. Now, as I'm getting older, I'm really pretty disabled. Over the years I think my main reaction has been to get discouraged over the never-ending struggle to control something I couldn't—that's real powerlessness. I've had lots of fear about what I'd be like in the end, and how soon I'd get that way. I've had lots of times you might call despairing, but I've always had to seem 'up' and show that I could cope. And I always knew, inside of me, that nobody understood—that's real loneliness. Then I'd go into remission and hope would spring up, but there was always fear with it—when would the other shoe drop again? It always has and always will."

Over the years Jane tried many different kinds of help—various kinds of therapy, bits and pieces of Eastern and Western religions. Each of them seemed useful for a little while, but nothing lasted. Jane drifted. Her spiritual life had no direction.

"I got into pills, painkillers. I was a mess, and ended up in AA. I worked at it, just the way I'd worked at things in the past. At that point in my life, though, after all that I'd been through, I didn't expect much. But there was this idea of my own Higher Power. I really did find this tremendous White Light inside of myself, and I really did turn myself over to it. What did I have to lose? Changes started, and they held. I'm convinced they held because my Light is really never-ending. It fills me with its energy, and my exhaustion lifts. My grandmother used to talk about seeing the light. I guess this is it."

Dan's Story

When Dan's heart disease was diagnosed, he was furious. Threatened by the possibility of a shortened life, he raged at the limitations his doctor put on him. He had to quit smoking, lose thirty pounds, stop eating hamburgers, fried potatoes, and "real" ice cream. And walk a mile a day? He was a busy man—where in hell could he find time? Dan was in a box; he could change his ways or he could die—and he didn't want to do either one. So he raged, and he blamed, and he lashed out at his family, friends, and doctor. And often, when he least expected it, fear would come, and he'd break out in a cold sweat and his hands would shake.

Then Dan's brother-in-law, a recovering alcoholic, suggested Dan go with him to an AA meeting. When Dan shouted, "That AA stuff is religious pap," his brother-in-law countered, "You're a mess; nobody can stand you— what have you got to lose?" So Dan went.

"What hooked me was the calmness of the meetings. People talked about the most intimate stuff, yet it was almost impersonal—I'd never seen anything like it. God was irrelevant to me, so the program itself became my Higher Power. Now, my life is very, very different. The doctor claims my blood pressure's down because of diet and exercise and medication, but I know that those things by themselves wouldn't have worked. It's the program that's taken away my rage and fear. The only medicine for those feelings was what you might call 'hanging out with my Higher Power.'"

The Little Red Book tells us that as a result of Step Three, five things can happen:

1. We surrender our self-centeredness.
2. We relax.
3. We avoid confusing the spiritual growth of the Twelve Step program with religion.
4. We do not try to define God.
5. We recognize and attempt to develop our spiritual possibilities.

As we work Step Three, we may begin to experience oneness with our Higher Power, and that can have great value for us. As Judith Viorst writes in her book *Necessary Losses,* "Experience of oneness can give us a respite from the solitude of separateness. And experiences of oneness can help us transcend our former limits, can help us grow."

Step Three: Written Exercise

1. How did working the First and Second Steps get you ready for Step Three?
2. List your resistances to turning over your will and life to your Higher Power, and then rank them in order of how important they are to you.
3. Take the resistances you listed above and write what's positive and negative about each one.
4. What do you think the outcome of turning your life and will over to a Higher Power could be?
5. How would you explain the statement "Becoming dependent on your Higher Power is really a way of becoming free"?
6. What do you think is meant by the statement "Even if your ideas of your Higher Power are not clear, that's all right. What's necessary is that you believe in the process"?

Step Three: Imagery Exercise

Close your eyes and imagine that you are alone, surrounded by some kind of barrier—a fence, a wall, a sheet of rigid plastic, glass panels like a greenhouse, whatever comes into your mind. The barrier is there because you have your disability or illness. You can't get out from behind it, and no one else can get in. Allow yourself to feel all the feelings you have about being alone, separated, and surrounded. Take time and let the feelings come, even the ones you almost never let yourself feel. Just for this moment it's safe to let them be there.

Ask your Higher Power to come to you. Ask it to help you. Allow yourself to feel surrounded by the caring your Higher Power gives you. Perhaps it holds you in its arms; perhaps something happens that is, for you, a sign that your Higher Power is there; perhaps you simply feel surrounded by its light and warmth. Whatever form it takes, the care is yours.

Next, taking your Higher Power with you, walk through the barrier that separates you from the world. Notice what happens as you pass through it. Notice the feeling you have as you get beyond it. Hold the feeling.

Now open your eyes. Quietly sit and hold the feeling of caring you received from your Higher Power and the strength you felt as you moved through the barrier. Carry this feeling with you as you return to your normal daily activities.

CHAPTER SIX

Taking an Inventory

Step Four: Made a searching and fearless moral inventory of ourselves.

The Fourth Step asks us to expose harmful emotions and character traits, to change them in a way that ensures our spiritual development. In the first two Steps we admitted that we need help and that there is a Power greater than ourselves available to help us. With the Third Step we turned our will and our lives over to that Higher Power.

The first three Steps are only the beginning of our journey toward spiritual fulfillment. Alone, they aren't enough. We are still insulated from serenity and peace. We are still trapped in our self-centeredness, false pride, and dishonesty. Concern with our physical problems, emotional pain, and denial interferes with our mental powers, and in many cases, has brought about irrational thoughts and behaviors.

All of this can result in extreme mental and physical hardship for us, and anxiety and suffering for others. Our lives will not improve until we deal with the negatives that inhibit our growth: the powerlessness, fear and anxiety, isolation and shame, anger and rage, blame and ambiguity, jealousy, grief, and exhaustion.

The main roadblock is denial. For those of us with

chronic illness or disability, denial is one of our most effective survival techniques. It protects us from more emotional pain than we can tolerate. But while denial drives our pain out of consciousness, it cannot erase that pain from our unconscious mind. The paradox is that while denial protects us from conscious hurt, it also keeps us from finding, facing, and ultimately releasing our negative emotions. In other words, it keeps us from the self-awareness that is the key to spiritual growth.

To defeat denial, we must find a way to recognize, meet, and understand that which is denied—in this case our emotional pain. We do this first by accepting our pain, then coming to understand what it means to us, and then finally receiving the help of our Higher Power. The objective of the Fourth Step is to overcome denial, to become clearly aware of our emotions and behaviors. Then we will be able to release our pain and use the energy it consumed for positive, spirit-enhancing changes.

Finding and Facing Our Pain

As we begin the Fourth Step, it is helpful to think about the many varied personalities we bring to it. Some of us are fairly flexible; it's quite easy for us to accept and assimilate new or different ideas. Some of us have personalities that are more set; it is harder, or takes longer, for us to incorporate changes in thinking. Some of us are what psychologists call "concrete" thinkers; we define things in terms of black and white, good and bad, right and wrong. Some of us think more abstractly; our view of things is more complicated. Some of us are older, with more life experience, some younger, with less living behind us. And some of us are fortunate enough to be blessed with high self-esteem, while others are less sure of their personal worth.

Having one or another kind of personality pattern is neither good nor bad. Such patterns are descriptions, not judgments. But each of us does have particular characteristics. When we begin the Fourth Step, it is helpful to take an honest look at how our personalities are organized. Realistic acceptance of how our mind works will start to break down our denial and open the way to true self-awareness.

When we became ill or disabled, we each had a personality with which we met our situation, and we each brought our unique personality to the Twelve Step program. To a great degree, these individual personality patterns will decide how we engage in our spiritual journey. They determine which of us are more controlled by rage and which by despair. They decide which of us more easily overcome feelings of powerlessness and which are locked in a seemingly unbreakable cycle of grief. But no matter who we are; or how we think, the process will work. The crucial thing is to find and face our negative attitudes, our "character defects," and our pain. We must commit ourselves to exposing these things and to accept the help of our Higher Power as we do so.

"What do you mean by 'find my pain'?" Meg asks. "Obviously I feel it, or I wouldn't try so hard to overcome it."

We do often feel the emotional pain attached to our condition. The very intensity of our need to manage it is a measure of our need to deny it. And the need to deny it comes from fear. We are afraid that if we look at it, if we allow ourselves to experience it, it will be more real; it will become worse. The truth is that rarely in life can something be made worse by accepting its existence. To the contrary, accepting its reality is the only way to begin to work through, or release, or change the situation or emotion. Unfortunately, what we often do is look at the painful event or feeling and then quickly turn away because we are so afraid of it. We become afraid not only of the pain but also of the fear. The cycle deepens and our protective denial builds. Working the Fourth Step can change this.

What follows in chapter 7 is an inventory of the major kinds of emotional pain connected with chronic illness or disability. The objective is to look at a certain emotional feeling, become familiar with it, and, consequently, reduce our fear of it. Our job is to remove feelings from the dark places where they live and bring them into the full light of familiarity.

CHAPTER SEVEN

Pain to Be Found and Faced

Powerlessness

A young woman with multiple sclerosis says, "I picture myself as a broken leaf on a fast-running stream, twirling around, being sucked under and then pulled back up to the surface. I am completely at the mercy of the water." A middle-aged diabetic is having increasing trouble with his vision. An older woman with moderate heart disease can easily care for herself and can do many things to slow down the progress of her illness.

The degree of impairment is very different for these people, yet they all know that the results of their disease are not within the limits of their control; they all suffer from feelings of powerlessness.

To feel powerlessness is a strong, debilitating, natural response to chronic illness or disability. We feel powerless because we *are* powerless—powerless to make our condition go away, powerless to be "normal," powerless over whatever has happened to our bodies, powerless over the final outcome. This leads to many other feelings—rage, panic, despair, lack of self-worth, anxiety, and on and on. The behaviors that grow out of feelings of powerlessness are unhealthy and self-destructive. They are manipulation, passive aggression, helplessness, lashing out at those around us, isolation of ourselves, expectation of failure, just plain giving up, and so many more. Being caught in the pain of powerlessness is like being caught in a whirlpool—it pulls us deeper and deeper into the vortex. We go round and round, and there seems to be no way out.

But there is a way, and again we're dealing with a paradox. We can lose the pain created by feelings of powerlessness by accepting powerlessness as our reality. This is the bedrock of the Twelve Step program; and once we agree to it, we can begin to use the Steps for our spiritual recovery.

When we admit to powerlessness we become humble, and humility can give us the power of freedom. We are freed from false pride, from grandiosity, and from the terrible tensions they can produce. We are our true selves, not trying to live up to tightly held unrealistic expectations. We are freed from the pressure of sparring with others as we try to manage their perceptions of us. From humility we learn that we may feel powerless and still have a busy, active, stimulating, and involved life. We can have rich relationships with family and friends, contribute to our community, and have a fulfilling spiritual life. To be able to do all this while accepting our powerlessness means that we are beyond being threatened by life. To truly accept powerlessness and to go on with living is to find serenity.

But many of us have been taught that powerlessness is bad. It is perceived as such a negative that we may turn and run from it. Thus, we may never fully come to understand our powerlessness, explore its positive possibilities, or learn to be comfortable with its negatives. Our job while working the Fourth Step is to examine and understand the many facets of our powerlessness—without fear and without running away. The exercises that follow can help. The imagery exercise is designed to help us examine and become thoroughly familiar with that feeling we call powerlessness, and the written exercise can help us see the place of powerlessness in everyday living.

Imagery Exercise to Find and Face Powerlessness

In your mind, let a symbol appear or a feeling arise that represents your powerlessness. The image could appear as a limp rag doll, the sensation of being lost, a leaf floating in the wind, or a feeling of struggling in a swampy morass. You might see yourself as trussed up in a rope or naked and shivering with cold. Whatever the image is, look at it or sense it very carefully. Take time to really see it, to really feel it. Don't hurry this or be afraid—the symbol is in your imagination and can't harm you.

Ask your powerlessness to tell you exactly what it is afraid of. Listen to its answer. Don't interrupt, or argue, or try to make it feel better. Just listen.

Ask your powerlessness what it has to offer you. Simply accept its answer quietly, no matter what it says, whether or not you approve, whether or not you agree, and no matter how strange it may seem.

Ask your powerlessness what it needs from you. Again, just listen.

Next, tell your powerlessness what it has meant to you, how it has helped you, how it has hurt.

As soon as you complete this conversation, write down what you have learned about your relationship with the part of you that feels powerless.

Repeat this exercise every day until the idea of powerlessness becomes familiar and raises less tension and fewer negative feelings.

Written Exercise to Help Deal with Powerlessness

1. Describe a specific circumstance that makes you feel powerless. Explain exactly how you feel in the situation. List as many feelings as you can.
2. Describe, in detail, what you usually do to relieve the pain of powerlessness in that particular circumstance.
3. Think of your response in terms of the first three Steps of the Twelve Step program. Describe how your thinking and behavior might be different if you followed those Steps.

Repeat this exercise for as many circumstances as you can think of that lead you to feeling powerless.

Fear and Anxiety

When I have the inner strength to face my fear, I will not send it outward as hatred or anger, or jealousy, or grief, or isolate myself because of it.

—Touchstones

Fear is a natural human reaction to an unfamiliar or threatening situation. It is physiological, sending messages to our brain that lead us to fight or flee. We are threatened and choose to stand and battle the menace, or we decide that absence is the better part of good sense and we leave. Sometimes when we are afraid, we simply acknowledge our reaction as fear. At other times we are afraid and hide it under another emotion. I am afraid someone may hurt me in physical therapy, so I defend myself by lashing out in anger at the therapist. I am afraid that my blindness will keep me from a job promotion, so I am jealous or resentful of my sighted competitor. I am afraid of how people react to my being in a wheelchair, so I isolate myself, cutting myself off from family and friends.

President Franklin Roosevelt gave us a key to spiritual growth when he said, "The only thing we have to fear is fear itself." Without fear, we can look at life with anticipation, finding our own way. If we are not afraid of how others view our illness or disability, we will not blame them or isolate ourselves; we can be enriched by life around us. If we are not afraid of the outcome of our condition, we can let go of grief—we can live each day to its fullest. When we face our fears and release them, our energy can be used to join with others instead of to fight, or flee, or fuel another negative emotion. Our immune systems will not be impaired by the overproduction of stress hormones. We will be mentally healthier and more physically sound.

Because fear is a natural physiological response, it will always reappear. So we need to understand the fearful part of ourselves; we need to discover its strengths as well as its weaknesses. Then when fear comes, we will know how to work with it so that it can be helpful and transitory instead of hurtful and controlling. Finding and facing our fear are central to our spiritual journey.

Imagery Exercise to Find and Face Fear or Anxiety

In your mind, let a symbol appear or a feeling arise that represents your fear or anxiety. Fear may appear as a dark, cloaked figure. Fear also often represents itself as a mass of blood or a writhing snake. You might see anxiety as a white field covered with squirming purple lines. Whatever the image is, look at it or sense it very carefully. Take time to really see it, to really feel it. Don't hurry this or be afraid—the symbol is in your imagination and can't harm you.

Ask yourself exactly what you are afraid of. Listen to the answer.

Ask your fear what it has to offer you. Simply accept its answer quietly, no matter what it says, whether or not you approve, whether or not you agree, and no matter how strange it may seem.

Ask your fear what it needs from you. Again, just listen.

Next, tell your fear what it has meant to you, how it has hurt you, how it has helped.

As soon as you complete this conversation, write down what you have learned about your relationship with the part of yourself that is fearful or anxiety-ridden.

Repeat this exercise every day until the idea of fear raises less tension and fewer negative feelings.

Written Exercise to Help Deal with Fear or Anxiety

1. Describe a specific circumstance that makes you feel fearful or anxious. Explain exactly how you feel in the situation. List as many feelings as you can.
2. Describe, in detail, what you usually do to relieve the pain of fear or anxiety in that particular circumstance.
3. Think of your response in terms of the first three Steps of the Twelve Step program. Describe how your thinking and behavior might be different if you followed those Steps.

Repeat this exercise for as many circumstances as you can think of that lead you to feeling fearful or anxious.

Isolation

I isolate myself because I'm ashamed, ashamed of how I look, ashamed of my weakness. When I'm around other people, I'm so self-conscious—I can never forget that I'm different.
—Sally, who has a disfigured arm

Sally was born with a shortened left arm that has no hand. Like many chronically ill or disabled people, she is ashamed and isolates herself because of her disability. Shame is a paralyzing emotion. It says, "I am a mistake, the damage is beyond repair, and the only thing is to re-ject myself and the world." Sally believes this.

"I isolate myself because I don't want to have to explain myself to others, and when I'm out in public, I feel like I always have to keep up a good front. The only time I don't have to do any explaining or keeping up is when I'm alone." This kind of isolation comes from being overly involved in others' reactions to our chronic illness or disability. We try to imagine what is happening in someone else's head and respond to it, instead of staying centered in our self.

As she ages, Ellen, whose life is increasingly limited by debilitating osteoarthritis, says, "I isolate myself because no one else can understand me." Some chronically ill or disabled people remain isolated in order to wallow in self-pity. Others act like martyrs, using their isolation as a tool of power to manipulate. And some angry people barricade themselves in isolation, taking the position of, "No one understands, so it's me against the world."

No matter what our reason, we will never gain spiritual health by holding on to isolation. Maybe it's possible for the spirits of monks and mystics to grow in solitude, but they aren't ordinary people. For most of us, remaining apart denies our human need for sociability and intimacy and decreases our self-esteem. Self-esteem can't rise when we know we aren't making a contribution to our family or community.

It's hard to find positive effects from the pain of isolation, but there are possibilities. As long as isolation does not become a permanent emotional style, living through it can give us a sense of security and competence. We know we can survive on our own. Also, it is possible to come out of a period of isolation with a strong sense of enjoyment of self. When we are content with ourselves, the time we spend apart from others changes from sad loneliness to joyful solitude. Finally, facing the misery of the isolated part of ourselves can lead to a loving self-nurturance that raises our self-esteem and leads us to honest relationships with other people.

But all of the positive outcomes of isolation are dependent on one thing—coming out of it. Becoming content solely with our own company may cripple us with complacency, and nurturing our misery can lead us further into ourselves. We need to learn to leave our isolation behind.

To do this, we first need to understand what keeps us where we are: Is it shame? The impossibility of always keeping up a front? Feelings of being misunderstood? Or any of a myriad of other reasons? The reasons will be different, depending on our unique personalities and life circumstances. We can act "as if" we enjoy getting together with other people; we can physically join the crowd; but until we understand our loneliness and isolation, we will feel the consequences. The key is to examine our loneliness, to find the reasons that we isolate ourselves or feel isolated from others. Once we understand, meaningful action can follow.

Imagery Exercise to Find and Face Isolation

In your mind, let a symbol appear or a feeling arise that represents your isolation. Isolation can present itself as a desert, a huge snowfield, or a lonely, shrouded figure. You might see yourself locked in a clear plastic box. Whatever the image is, look at it or sense it very carefully. Take time to really see it, to really feel it. Don't hurry this or be afraid—the symbol is in your imagination and can't harm you.

Ask your isolation to tell you exactly what it is afraid of. Listen to its answer. Don't interrupt or argue. Just listen.

Ask your isolation what it has to offer you. Simply accept its answer quietly, no matter what it says, whether or not you approve, whether or not you agree, and no matter how strange it may seem.

Ask your isolation what it needs from you. Again, just listen.

Next, tell your isolation what it has meant to you, how it has hurt you, how it has helped.

As soon as you complete this conversation, write down what you have learned about your relationship with the part of yourself that feels isolated.

Repeat this exercise every day until the idea of isolation raises less tension and fewer negative feelings.

Written Exercise to Help Deal with Isolation

1. Describe a specific circumstance that makes you feel isolated. Explain exactly how you feel in the situation. List as many feelings as you can.
2. Describe, in detail, what you usually do to relieve the pain of isolation in that particular circumstance.

3. Think of your response in terms of the first three Steps of the Twelve Step program. Describe how your thinking and behavior might be different if you followed those Steps.

Repeat this exercise for as many circumstances as you can think of that lead you to feeling isolated.

Anger and Rage

Powerlessness may be my basic fear, but it is this anger that's going to kill me.
—Fred, who has hypertension

Fred struggles with extremely high blood pressure; for him, anger can be deadly. When anger is directed outward, toward other people, it can turn them away from us, and we become isolated. Then we typically use our leftover emotional energy to rationalize our angry behavior. But rationalization is a conscious process; our unconsciousness isn't fooled. It knows we have behaved badly, and our self-esteem shrivels as our self-hatred grows. If we are the kind of personality that handles anger by turning it inward, it can cause apathy, immobility, and depression. This, too, results in isolation and can block out any joy, contentment, satisfaction, or peace that we might otherwise feel.

On the other hand, anger focused at a specific, realistic target is a strong, useful human response to fear. If we can put aside unrealistic mental battles, we can use the energy of anger to move us toward our goals.

Instead of projecting his anger outward by screaming at his physical therapist, or inward by refusing to cooperate, John, a young amputee, realistically focuses it on his situation and uses his angry energy to learn to walk. "I hate all this; I won't be a cripple. Just watch me walk now—and by God, I'll go farther tomorrow."

Mary, who has been diagnosed with a rare form of leukemia, feels at one moment like screaming at her husband and children and at the next like sitting in a closet and crying. Instead, she goes to the university medical library to learn all she can about her disease in order to take a more active role in her treatment.

Ellen, seventy-seven, has recently become wheelchair-bound by osteoporosis (a condition characterized by decrease in bone mass). She overcomes her inertia, turns off the daytime television that is meaningless to her, and registers for an introductory class in computers.

Each of these people has found his or her own way to use the energy of anger. Each has learned not to displace it onto others or direct it inward, but to use it as fuel for emotional and spiritual growth.

A special relationship exists between anger and the Twelve Step program, particularly with the First and Second Steps. Most chronically ill or disabled people are angry. There are overt ragers, covert manipulators, and people who don't feel angry but are depressed—all from fighting the pain of powerlessness. As we take the First Step, we stop fighting and stop trying to prove that we are in total control of our lives—we are led to accept our powerlessness and become humble. Humility and rage don't go together. We take the Second Step and gain hope that one day we will be healed from the scars of anger. Now, with Step Four, we prepare to do our part. We will find and face the ball of rage inside of us. We will search out its hiding places, so that ultimately we can use our anger constructively or let it go.

Imagery Exercise to Find and Face Anger and Rage

In your mind, let a symbol appear or a feeling arise that represents your anger or rage. Many people find some form of fire, the color red, or perhaps a huge wall that blocks off vision. Whatever the image is, look at it or sense it very carefully. Take time to really see it, to really feel it. Don't hurry this or be afraid—the symbol is in your imagination and can't harm you.

Ask your anger or rage to tell you exactly what it is afraid of. Listen to its answer. Don't interrupt or argue. Just listen.

Ask your anger or rage what it has to offer you. Simply accept its answer quietly, no matter what it says, whether or not you approve, whether or not you agree, and no matter how strange it may seem.

Ask your anger or rage what it needs from you. Again, just listen.

Next, tell your anger or rage what it has meant to you, how it has hurt you, how it has helped.

As soon as you complete this conversation, write down what you have learned about your relationship with the part of yourself that is angry.

Repeat this exercise every day until the idea of anger or rage raises less tension and fewer negative feelings.

Written Exercise to Help Deal with Anger and Rage

1. Describe a specific circumstance that makes you feel anger or rage. Explain exactly how you feel in the situation. List as many feelings as you can.
2. Describe, in detail, what you usually do to relieve the pain of anger or rage in that particular circumstance.
3. Think of your response in terms of the first three Steps of the Twelve Step program. Describe how your thinking and behavior might be different if you followed those Steps.

Repeat this exercise for as many circumstances as you can think of that lead you to feeling anger or rage.

Ambiguity and Blame

Almost the worst thing about this whole situation is that I can't make sense out of it. Why did it happen? Why me? What's the point? Who do I blame?

—Anne, twenty-one, quadriplegic from a diving accident

Having a chronic illness or disability places us in an ambiguous situation. We can't figure out why things are as they are, what it all means, or what to do about it. As we struggle to make sense of our illness or disability, we often turn to blame.

John, a man facing complicated heart surgery, says, "My wife certainly could have done more to help. She wasn't very good at working out the doctor's diet—and, after all, she's the cook."

Elaine has just found out she has lung cancer. She is struggling to understand her treatment options and the "why" of her illness: "Why? Why didn't I listen when everyone told me to quit smoking? I might have prevented this. I was so strong-minded and dumb that I guess I deserve what I've gotten."

For most people, being put in an ambiguous, negative situation leads to panic. We can't make sense out of it; we are unbalanced and want an immediate and simple answer. The easiest way to find that answer and give meaning to the situation is to blame. Blaming is almost reflex, whether we blame others or ourselves.

But blame is rarely useful; it almost always needs denial to maintain it. When we blame, denial controls our reactions and makes our decisions. Blaming leads to other hurtful consequences too. John, the heart patient who blames his wife, makes her feel guilty. Her anger rises up to match his own, and the possibilities of their working out a cooperative postsurgical relationship are diminished. As a consequence, John's future is jeopardized. Elaine's self-hatred results in depression that impairs decision making about her choices of treatment. It also impairs the function of her immune system, undermining whatever treatment she and her doctors finally decide on.

But there is an important positive effect from finding and facing the emotional pain of ambiguity and blame. We can learn to accept ambiguity as normal, face it calmly, study the situation from all sides, and ask for help from our Higher Power. Then we can rationally assess responsibility. We do this by learning to recognize where responsibility lies without adding the emotional negatives of charging error or fault, without leaping into blame. As a result, we can be released from denial, develop clarity in viewing our lives, and make responsible decisions. We can also become secure in our ability to face ambiguity. We can face our future calmly knowing that emotional pain and blame no longer control us.

Imagery Exercise to Find and Face Ambiguity and Blame

In your mind, let a symbol appear or a feeling arise that represents your feelings of ambiguity and blame. Perhaps you will see a fork in the road ahead of you, or maybe you will get a sense of being in a dense fog. Whatever the image is, look at it or sense it very carefully. Take time to really see it, to really feel it. Don't hurry this or be afraid—the symbol is in your imagination and can't harm you.

Ask your ambiguity and blame to tell you exactly what they are afraid of. Listen to their answer. Don't interrupt or argue. Just listen.

Ask your ambiguity and blame what they have to offer you. Simply accept their answer quietly, no matter what they say, whether or not you approve, whether or not you agree, and no matter how strange it may seem.

Ask your ambiguity and blame what they need from you. Again, just listen.

Next, tell your ambiguity and blame what they have meant to you, how they have hurt you, how they have helped.

As soon as you complete this conversation, write down what you have learned about your relationship with the part of yourself that feels ambiguous and blameful.

Repeat this exercise every day until the idea of ambiguity and blame raises less tension and fewer negative feelings.

Written Exercise to Help Deal with Ambiguity and Blame

1. Describe a specific circumstance that makes you feel ambiguous or makes you want to blame others. Explain exactly how you feel in the situation. List as many feelings as you can.
2. Describe, in detail, what you usually do to relieve the pain of ambiguity and blame in that particular circumstance.
3. Think of your response in terms of the first three Steps of the Twelve Step program. Describe how your thinking and behavior might be different if you followed those Steps.

Repeat this exercise for as many circumstances as you can think of that lead you to feeling ambiguous or blameful.

Jealousy

It's funny, before the accident I used to like to read, and I liked studying too. Now I couldn't care less about that stuff—all I think about is what I can't do. It's like when I watch football on TV. I really hate those guys, because they can play and I will never be on the field again.

—Dave, paralyzed in a motorcycle accident

Dave, nineteen, is paraplegic and is wheelchair-bound for life. He used to enjoy reading, thinking, and talking about ideas with his friends and family. Now he thinks about how he hates the people involved in the freewheeling physical activities that he is denied. Jealousy—and its partners, envy and resentment—form a painful, ugly trinity. This trio can separate us from others and deny us intimacy. There is simply no way to combine intimacy with envy or resentment or jealousy.

When we are jealous, we focus on our weaknesses rather than on our strengths. We think about what we don't have instead of what we do. We think about what others have that we don't. We are apt to define things as negative rather than positive. We may look outside of ourselves for gratification, rather than inside. When we are jealous, we often reject opportunities for positive and spiritually enhancing experiences.

Dave, the young paraplegic, refuses to meet with a teacher who wants to talk with him about tutoring a student who is failing Spanish: "It's a stupid idea—I help him raise his average so next year he can play varsity basketball when I can't."

Dave's jealousy has led him to shallow-mindedness and mean thinking.

Jealousy also can lead to obsession and increasingly narrows the limits of our thoughts.

Since her mastectomy five years ago, Carol has been unable to decide whether or not to have her breast reconstructed. "I find myself noticing other women's breasts all the time. It's crazy, but I can't help it. And when I see a woman with nice ones, I hate her. I wish her bad things. That's crazy too. I'm not a mean or vindictive person, but I'm so jealous I just feel nuts."

Carol is so completely tied up in her jealousy of other women that she can't realistically relate to her own situation. Her thinking whirls in narrow, obsessive circles.

The emotional pain of jealousy is hard to change, because we often don't recognize it. We feel jealous, or resentful, or envious, and try to get over it by arguing with ourselves. We try to use reason to counteract unyielding emotion. This rarely works. If we look beneath the grinding pain of jealousy, envy, or resentment, we usually find that the underlying pain is an all-encompassing sadness.

Finding our jealousy and facing the more basic pain beneath it gives us the chance to understand our deep sadness and insecurity. This understanding focuses our healing on basic hurts, rather than on the secondary pains of the ugly trinity. Then we can ask our Higher Power for help, our spirit can grow, and we can take another step toward serenity.

Imagery Exercise to Find and Face Jealousy

In your mind, let a symbol appear or a feeling arise that represents your jealousy. A common symbol for jealousy is the color green: Sometimes it can be a field of color or sometimes an object. Whatever the image is, look at it or sense it very carefully. Take time to really see it, to really feel it. Don't hurry this or be afraid—the symbol is in your imagination and can't harm you.

Ask your jealousy to tell you exactly what it is afraid of. Listen to its answer. Don't interrupt or argue. Just listen.

Ask your jealousy what it has to offer you. Simply accept its answer quietly, no matter what it says, whether or not you approve, whether or not you agree, and no matter how strange it may seem.

Ask your jealousy what it needs from you. Again, just listen.

Next, tell your jealousy what it has meant to you, how it has hurt you, how it has helped.

As soon as you complete this conversation, write down what you have learned about your relationship with the part of yourself that is jealous.

Repeat this exercise every day until the idea of jealousy raises less tension and fewer negative feelings.

Written Exercise to Help Deal with Jealousy

1. Describe a specific circumstance that makes you feel jealous. Explain exactly how you feel in the situation. List as many feelings as you can.

2. Describe, in detail, what you usually do to relieve the pain of jealousy in that particular circumstance.

3. Think of your response in terms of the first three Steps of the Twelve Step program. Describe how your thinking and behavior might be different if you followed those Steps.

Repeat this exercise for as many circumstances as you can think of that lead you to feeling jealous.

Grief

When I was in it, there was no way I could have sorted it out. You just don't realize that grief has taken over your life—and you can't understand what's happened to you until it's over. Getting back to normal is the only way to put it—during that time I was absolutely not myself. Now I'd say I'm normal, but I'm not the same person I was before it all happened.

—Jean, amputee

Grief is a natural response to the onset of chronic illness or a disabling accident. The process of grieving, however, will be different for everyone. It depends on the nature and severity of the condition and on the personality of the grieving person. The pattern of the disease will also make a difference. An illness with recurring remissions often keeps a person cycling through the same phases of grief, and a relentlessly debilitating disease means there are ever-increasing losses to assimilate. A child disabled at birth may grieve periodically as she recognizes how the disability affects her life. Grief can be triggered on entering school, becoming a teenager, and moving into adult-hood. As the disabled woman matures, she puts together the emotional and psychological skills and strengths learned from the losses experienced during childhood and adolescence. Now, in adulthood, the changes may not come so quickly. Finally, there is time to resolve what-ever grief she may still attach to her disability.

Grief is an emotional process that can take over our lives. It can control our relationships, our lifestyles, and our decisions. Researchers who study grief tell us that di-rectly after any important loss—whether it's a divorce, re-tirement, death of a loved one, or the onset of a chronic illness or disability—we shouldn't make major decisions or plan radical changes in our lives. They say that to do so is foolish, because our judgment is clouded and con-trolled by our grieving.

As difficult as it is to accept, grief is a protective mech-anism for the mind. In the beginning it is a purely emo-tional reaction; intellect has little or no impact on it. In the first phase of grief, we use disbelief and denial to block out the seemingly unbearable fact of our illness or dis-ablement—perhaps our mind needs to rest and gather strength to face the emotional storms to come.

Five years ago, Jean lost her hand in a factory accident. "When this first happened, I kept telling myself to face reality. Your hand is gone. It's gone. You'll never have it back or be the same. But I just couldn't feel anything; my mind was numb."

The second phase of grief acts as an emotional catharsis in which we bring feelings to the surface. These feelings can range from rage to disbelief. Jean explains what happened to her:

"When it hit, it hit with a fury. My emotions were wild, all over the map. They flipped around so fast and were so strong that I was sure I was going crazy."

But she wasn't crazy; she was just grieving. As we slowly move through this phase, our emotionally unbalanced system begins to right itself. Little by little, with many regressions, rationality and calm begin to reappear.

In the final phase of grief, we regain our psychological balance. We have a new definition of self, forged in the turmoil we have been through. We now become prepared to live life in terms of this new self-image. Jean relates her experience:

"I would never have asked for this to happen to me—and I will probably always wish it hadn't. But it has. What is, is. And in the process I've become a much stronger—probably a much wiser—person."

The resolution of grief is crucial to our spiritual health. As we work back and forth through the stages, our spirit evolves and real personal and emotional change can happen. Through grieving, we can learn to admit our powerlessness and accept reality. We can let go of the past, ourselves as we were, our goals, our hopes and dreams. We begin to live honestly in today's situation, without denial, and we set new goals and dream new dreams appropriate to our current reality. We feel released, at peace with ourselves and with our world.

Imagery Exercise to Find and Face Grief

In your mind, let a symbol appear or a feeling arise that represents your grief. Grief might take the form of a deep pit or a rolling black cloud. Many people see a shrouded figure, standing alone. Whatever the image is, look at it or sense it very carefully. Take time to really see it, to really feel it. Don't hurry this or be afraid—the symbol is in your imagination and can't harm you.

Ask your grief to tell you exactly what it is afraid of. Listen to its answer. Don't interrupt or argue. Just listen.

Ask your grief what it has to offer you. Simply accept its answer quietly, no matter what it says, whether or not you approve, whether or not you agree, and no matter how strange it may seem.

Ask your grief what it needs from you. Again, just listen.

Next, tell your grief what it has meant to you, how it has hurt you, how it has helped.

As soon as you complete this conversation, write down what you have learned about your relationship with the part of yourself that is grieving.

Repeat this exercise every day until the idea of grief raises less tension and fewer negative feelings.

Written Exercise to Help Deal with Grief

1. Describe a specific circumstance that makes you feel grief. Explain exactly how you feel in the situation. List as many feelings as you can.

2. Describe, in detail, what you usually do to relieve the pain of grief in that particular circumstance.

3. Think of your response in terms of the first three Steps of the Twelve Step program. Describe how your thinking and behavior might be different if you followed those Steps.

Repeat this exercise for as many circumstances as you can think of that lead you to feeling grief.

Exhaustion

One of the things that makes it so hard to deal with my arthritis is the sheer exhaustion that I feel. It's not depression; I'm just tired.
—Ellen, whose life is limited by painful and debilitating arthritis

The exhaustion that comes with chronic illness or disability is based on both physical and emotional fatigue. This is not the debility of depression or the totally empty feeling of deep despair, but a realistic reaction to physical and emotional exertion. Physically, our disabilities cause us to drain an excessive amount of energy from an already depleted body as we carry out the activities in everyday life. It simply takes more energy for a man with multiple sclerosis to walk down the stairs than it does for his healthy wife. For a stroke patient, or a person with cerebral palsy, eating uses a concentration of energy that most of us don't require as we maneuver knife and fork, moving food to our mouths.

Emotionally, our disabilities empty us too. We may be exhausted from experiencing or trying to control the emotional pain we attach to our condition. Sam, a man recently diagnosed with hypertension, says, "I don't know which wears me out more—the anger I feel about all of this or the emotional energy it takes to keep my blood pressure down." We may be worn out by raging against our powerlessness, by repressing or fighting our fear, by maintaining our rationalization and denial as we blame, or by the ferocious mood swings of grief. Because of the isolation so many of us experience, we are kept from being energized by relationships with friends and loved ones.

But there are lessons to be learned from exhaustion. We can learn how to care for our bodies. We can learn how to strengthen them and invigorate them with exercise. We can learn how to pace ourselves, to find our own unique physical limits. We can learn how to fuel our bodies with good food and learn which foods give energy and which ones steal it. We can learn how to renew ourselves with rest. We can learn when to rest, what's too much or too little. We can learn how to be aware of our bodies and keep our physical conditioning in perspective.

We gain the awareness of physical vulnerability earlier than most people do. For a chronically ill woman, the fatigue associated with aging doesn't come as a shock—she may not like what happens as she gets older, but she knows that her body is vulnerable to changes outside of her control.

Exhaustion can teach us to care for our mind too. We become depleted from living with emotional pain, but as we learn to find, face, and release this pain, we develop mental techniques that will be lifelong guides for feeling free and alive. In giving up efforts to control our pain, in working the Twelve Steps, in asking for help from our Higher Power, we lose uncertainty, confusion, and exhaustion. We find peace.

Imagery Exercise to Find and Face Exhaustion

In your mind, let a symbol appear or a feeling arise that represents your exhaustion. To many people, exhaustion appears as a sensation of nothingness. White or gray are often the associated colors. Whatever the image is, look at it or sense it very carefully. Take time to really see it, to really feel it. Don't hurry this or be afraid—the symbol is in your imagination and can't harm you.

Ask your exhaustion to tell you exactly what it is afraid of. Listen to its answer. Don't interrupt or argue. Just listen.

Ask your exhaustion what it has to offer you. Simply accept its answer quietly, no matter what it says, whether or not you approve, whether or not you agree, and no matter how strange it may seem.

Ask your exhaustion what it needs from you. Again, just listen.

Next, tell your exhaustion what it has meant to you, how it has hurt you, how it has helped.

As soon as you complete this conversation, write down what you have learned about your relationship with the part of yourself that feels exhausted.

Repeat this exercise every day until the idea of exhaustion raises less tension and fewer negative feelings.

Written Exercise to Help Deal with Exhaustion

1. Describe a specific circumstance that makes you feel exhausted. Explain exactly how you feel in the situation. List as many feelings as you can.
2. Describe, in detail, what you usually do to relieve the pain of exhaustion in that particular circumstance.
3. Think of your response in terms of the first three Steps of the Twelve Step program. Describe how your thinking and behavior might be different if you followed those Steps.

Repeat this exercise for as many circumstances as you can think of that lead you to feeling exhausted.

CHAPTER EIGHT

Consequences of Unfaced Pain

Living with the emotional pain we've been discussing has very specific psychological and behavioral consequences that we need to recognize before we can work toward a more rewarding life.

Denial—We pretend that our condition doesn't exist, or doesn't affect us to the degree that it really does, or that it will go away if we ignore it. In other words, we deny our own reality.

Dishonesty—We evade the truth of our condition when we relate to others. We use half-truths, distorted definitions, and constantly try to manage the impression we make.

Intolerance—We become so rigid in our need to control our environment and so centered on our problems that we become intolerant and critical of others.

Self-pity—Our elaborate self-concern causes us to resent and reject others. We see ourselves as central to our entire social universe and feel self-pity when others aren't as consumed with our problems as we are.

False pride—False pride is pride based on the opinion of others. It develops when we hide our weaknesses and vulnerabilities and reach for achievements and status that others will judge as superior. This is different from true pride, which is based on our own opinion of ourselves. We feel true pride when we are proud of an accomplishment because we have met our goals and have maintained our integrity. A stroke victim suffers false pride when she strives to walk so that others will see her as "normal." She feels true pride when she is able to walk fifteen steps and congratulates herself for overcoming the tremendous physical odds against her.

The consequences of emotional pain come from excessive self-involvement; yet, in seeming contradiction, they keep us alienated from ourselves. Our cycles of emotional pain separate us from our real self, the self we are trying to avoid, the self who is a normal person and who is chronically ill or disabled. Another devastating effect of denial, dishonesty, intolerance, self-pity, and false pride is that they keep us insulated from friendship and intimacy. Others may see our reality more clearly than we do; their vision is more objective. But in our pain and our need to control our environment, we refuse to ask for, or accept, the assessments of friends and loved ones. Much as they care about us, they feel like outsiders, and we feel safer if we keep it that way.

A particularly harmful consequence of unfaced pain is the way we may use our emotional pain itself to control others. We may explode with anger, forcing others to walk on eggshells when they are with us. Or we use mood swings as tools of power.

The mother of a seventeen-year-old quadriplegic son says, "His mood controls the mood of the whole family. If he's up, so are we. When he's depressed, we all feel awful and do anything we can to make him perk up."

Some of us become experts at using guilt to manipulate others. We get our way by making others sorry for us. Then, if they show their pity, we criticize them for making us feel "different."

Our friends and families are kept off balance; they aren't sure how to reach out to us. Some try to read our minds and accept our manipulative behavior. These people become martyrs or codependents who spend their time trying to figure out what we want without considering that it might be hurtful to them. Some give up, relating to us only superficially or avoiding us altogether. If we refuse to accept our reality as it truly is, if we continue to live within our cycles of pain, our friends and families are forced to leave us. Everyone loses—everyone is deprived of intimacy, warmth, and spiritual growth.

We don't have to live this way. Remember, our purpose in working the Fourth Step is to expose the harmful emotions and character traits that we have developed as a result of our physical condition—and to change them in a way that ensures our spiritual development. So far, we have made an inventory of our emotional pain; in Steps Five, Six, and Seven we will discover a way to change it. As we prepare to give up the feelings that can destroy our spirit, we need to briefly discuss the soul-enriching emotions with which we can replace them.

CHAPTER NINE

Filling the Void with Positives

Hope: The Mainspring of Our Life Force

Hope is like the sun which, as we journey toward it, casts the shadow of our burden behind us.

—Samuel Smiles

When we talk about spiritual fulfillment, we speak of love, serenity, faith, and joy. We often overlook hope, yet hope is crucial. Without it our spirit could not evolve. The old saying "Hope springs eternal in the human breast" is true. Hope is built into the psychological makeup of human beings; it's an integral part of us. We may take it for granted, but it's the mainspring of our life force. Hope is the energy that gets us up in the morning. It promotes enthusiasm, confidence, and joy. It lets us dream and set goals. Another saying tells us, "As long as there's life, there's hope." Many seriously ill people use this belief to sustain their spirits when there isn't much else to cling to. It also works the other way: "As long as there's hope, there's life." Doctors and their patients often believe that medical miracles are simply hope given physical form.

Some people give up hope, make a clear decision, and die. They say, "I'm ready to go now," and they do. Doctors and nurses who work with terminally ill patients know it's not unusual for a patient to die if he or she gives up hope. Religions based on black magic work this way too. People discover they are cursed, give up hope, turn their faces to the wall, and waste away. Psychologists cite case after case where clients lose hope and then lose their minds. And negative self-fulfilling prophecies work because they, too, steal hope.

Hope fuels our life force, but it needs to be applied realistically. This doesn't mean we shouldn't hope for the very best, but we can misuse hope when we use it to support denial. A man whose leukemia is in remission can hope that the remission will be a long one, but should not use it to believe he is cured. Rather, he must use the strength of hope to live his life as fully as he can, regardless of how long his disease is dormant. Hope may help his body stay as healthy as possible, and it can make him spiritually strong.

Love: Nurturing Another's Spiritual Growth

Love is the will to extend one's self for the purpose of nurturing one's own or another's spiritual growth.
—M. Scott Peck, *The Road Less Traveled*

What we choose to love is very important, for what we love leads our eyes, ears, and hearts on a pilgrimage that shapes the texture of our lives.
—Wayne Muller, *How, Then, Shall We Live?*

We don't usually think about love as an act of choice or will. We'd rather believe that it is happenstance, a feeling that descends on us from someplace or something, but that is not true. As any husband, wife, parent, lover, friend, caregiver, or person with a deep social conscience knows, love involves choice, intention, and action. To love is an act of one's will; we love when we choose to exert ourselves in the cause of spiritual growth. To will ourselves to love is to dedicate ourselves to the spirit.

Extending ourselves toward the spiritual growth of others can create the soul-fulfilling emotions of connection, intimacy, and true caring. It relieves our destructive self-centeredness and moves us out of ourselves into the human community. Sometimes our loving of others is perceived as supportive; we extend ourselves in ways that they like. This is the case when we care for the garden or the pets of a hospitalized friend. Sometimes our loving is perceived in a different way. An adolescent may have trouble understanding that his parents' insistence on remedial summer school is an act of love. But the bottom line is in the purpose. If the action is directed toward the nurturing of another's spiritual growth, it is love.

To extend ourselves toward our own spiritual growth is equally important—and that is what working the Twelve Step program does. This is a program of love designed to heal spiritual illness. When we choose the Twelve Steps as a guide, when we intend to work with them to rid ourselves of emotional pain, when we make them our way of living, we are nurturing our spiritual growth. We are loving ourselves.

Joy: Remaining Open to Its Possibilities

Joy is the life of man's life.
—Benjamin Whichcote, *Moral Aphorisms,* 1753

Joys do not abide, but take wing and fly away.
—Martial, *Epigrams*

Contentment, satisfaction, happiness—it's a wonderful moment when these good feelings surge up in us. Sometimes we plan for them. We set the stage, hoping to feel contented or satisfied, and we spend lots of time searching for whatever we call happiness. But joy is different. We can't create it. It's almost always unexpected. Pure joy is like a bursting light; it explodes and swells within us. And it's nearly always triggered by something spiritual. Joy is different from the exultation that comes from achievement or with the feeling of power. Exultation that comes from achievement can be soul-fulfilling if the achievement is a loving one, if we know that it is useful to ourselves and others. But there is danger that it may encourage us toward achievement for its own sake. The exultation that comes with the winning of power is most often soul-destructive. It kills humility as it reinforces our desire to win, to be superior, to hold others beneath us.

True joy doesn't happen often. It comes with a flash of instant recognition of life and of love: the clear elegance of a flower, the green glory of a spring day, the beauty of our sleeping child, the soaring of a Beethoven violin concerto. For the fleeting moment that it is with us, joy means total connection, connection with something greater than ourselves. In joy we connect with the universe. It is momentary, total spiritual fulfillment. We can't foresee joy, but if we remain open to its possibility, it will come.

Faith: The Miraculous Connection

Reason is our soul's left hand, Faith her right. By these we reach divinity.
—John Donne, *To the Countess of Bedford*

Since the beginning of time people have created many different names and ideologies to try to explain the inexplicable force that operates our universe. But no matter what the force has been called, no matter what rituals and institutions have been developed around it, for all time and for all people, one part of the process has been the same. That part of the process is the connection, the emotional relationship, between people and their life force—the connection we call faith.

One entity is the human being; the other, the life force. The life force can be called many things: God, Buddha, Allah, Higher Power, Love, Nature, White Light, and others. If the human being and the life force are to get together, the current that runs between them must be faith. It is faith that activates the system.

Many people walk through life oblivious to the potential of the life force that surrounds them. They just don't have the faith to connect with it. On the other hand, there are those whose lives are based on what Søren Kierkegaard, Danish philosopher and theologian, called the "leap of faith." A leap of faith occurs when people believe in a Power beyond themselves even when they cannot explain it or touch it.

From the time we are children, we hear that "faith can move mountains" or that "faith can make miracles." In real life, the combination of our Self, our Faith, and our Higher Power may not move mountains, but it can create miracles. Some of us will experience major miracles, the kind Bernie Siegel talks about in *Love, Medicine, and Miracles*. But for most of us, the miracles will be smaller. They will be unique, life-enriching experiences that will happen when we remain open to the possibilities in life and keep our faith turned on.

Serenity: Receiving Each Day's Joy

My greatest wealth is the deep stillness in which I strive and grow and win what the world cannot take from me with fire and sword.
—Goethe

We may often think of serenity as calmness, peace, tranquillity—a state of uninterrupted smoothness. To most of us, monks or Yogi meditators are examples of serene humans. A gently flowing stream reminds us of serenity in nature. To be serene can be interpreted as floating through life, and serenity is sometimes like this. We have calm, tranquil times and they are wonderful. But the serenity we seek as a result of our spiritual evolution is not a passive state. On the contrary, it is a very active one. It means engaging with life, experiencing it fully, yet not being burdened by it.

Medical researchers have taught us that there is a difference between "stress," which is a natural part of the human condition and which promotes energy, and "dis-stress," which means to be destroyed rather than energized by the pressures of life.

A fourth-grade teacher goes energetically through her day with twenty-five students. Her energy can be serene energy moving without pressure and with love, or it can be distressed energy fueled by impatience, frustration, and anger. The teacher experiences one set of circumstances but can respond serenely or with emotional turbulence.

To be serene is to live an average kind of life under sometimes stressful conditions without experiencing dis-stress.

Serenity is hard to come by. It requires that we surrender the outcome while we lovingly nurture and trust the process. We must stay present to the possibility of what each day offers and to receive its joy. For most of us, the way to accomplish this is by being deeply and consciously aware of the presence of the spiritual resources that surround us.

Spirit-Enhancing Emotions

In addition to love, hope, joy, faith, and serenity, there are many other positive, constructive emotions that will fill the void left by our released pain. Our spirit is nurtured when we feel the following:

accepted	competent	enthusiastic	proud
appreciated	complete	fulfilled	relaxed
assured	confident	intimate	satisfied
calm	connected	lovable	secure
cheerful	curious	loving	wanted
comfortable	delighted	optimistic	wonderful

We all know these feelings and others like them. They are natural emotions for everyone. Many of us with chronic illnesses or physical challenges have had them blocked out by our pain; now we need to encourage them. The more we feel them, the more they become our usual way of being, and the more our spirits will grow. The following two exercises can help.

Written Exercise to Encourage Spirit-Enhancing Emotions

1. Describe a specific circumstance that makes you feel _____. (Pick one of the feelings described or listed in this chapter.)
2. Describe circumstances or feelings that for you interfere with making you feel _____.
3. Think of your response as it relates to the first three Steps of the Twelve Step program and to the emotional pain discussed in the Fourth Step inventory. Describe how you might encourage your feeling of _____ if you use what you have learned.

Repeat this exercise for any of the spirit-enhancing emotions.

Imagery Exercise to Encourage Spirit-Enhancing Emotions

In your mind, let a symbol appear that represents a feeling mentioned in this chapter.

Look at it very carefully. Take time to see and feel it. Don't hurry this; let the feeling come.

Ask this feeling what it has to offer you. Simply accept its answer, no matter what it says.

Ask this feeling what it needs from you.

Next, tell this feeling what it means to you, how it helps you.

Finally, ask this feeling to return, again and again. Welcome it.

As soon as you complete this conversation, write down what you have learned from this exercise about your relationship with this feeling.

Repeat this exercise for any of the spirit-enhancing emotions you would like to feel more often.

CHAPTER TEN

Taking Our Struggle to the Outside World

Step Five: Admitted to the God of our understanding, to ourselves, and to another human being the exact nature of our wrongs.

In Step Four we made a searching and fearless inventory of ourselves. We examined the destructive and hurtful ways we have reacted to our illness or physical challenge. We discussed the wrong thinking and attitudes that have resulted in the emotional pain that keeps us from serenity.

Step Five is a turning point. As a result of the first four Steps, we have built the basis on which we can live a truly spiritual life, a life as our real selves. We have had an internal struggle, and now the Fifth Step asks that we take our struggle to the world outside of our own psyche. It requires that we admit the exact nature of our "wrongs," first to ourselves and our Higher Power and then to another human being. It makes the transition from thought to action, from intrapersonal to interpersonal, from aloneness to connection.

We carried out the first Steps inside of our heads. Now it is time to test our commitment to honesty and our willingness to face the consequences of our honesty. As we work Step Five, *The Little Red Book* promises us we will move from growth in spiritual beliefs to growth in spiritual experience.

Step Four may have been difficult for us. It was hard to break through our denial and resistance and admit that the pain described was the pain we felt. It was hard to look at old feelings and memories that we have spent much time and energy hiding from ourselves. It was hard to admit we behave in ways destructive to ourselves and others.

On the other hand, there is great benefit from this hard work. There is relief in admitting the reality of our emotional reactions, of making them our conscious partners. We always knew they were there; our subconscious wasn't fooled by whatever pretenses our conscious mind concocted. Our hurt is no longer secret, a specter to be hidden and ashamed of.

Step Five builds on Step Four and gives us the opportunity to complete the acknowledgment of our pain. We are asked to share the exact nature of our wrongs and the extent of our pain with ourselves so we can accept our darker side and thus live whole. We also share our wrongs with our Higher Power, which increases our trust in that relationship. Finally, we share those wrongs with another human being. This last part can be frightening. After all, we may have spent much of our time preventing others from seeing the feelings and emotions hidden inside us.

But when we carry out this Step, we have an experience that many of us didn't think was possible. When we open ourselves to another person, he or she will see our struggle, turmoil, nastiness, and aggression and not turn away. Instead of being repelled, he or she will listen and understand. To most people, this gives great release and relief; for some, it feels like a miracle.

Also, the Fifth Step gives us firsthand experience in the power of humility. We try so hard to feel powerful by keeping up a front, by controlling and managing the impression we make on others. Yet the humility required of us when we speak fully of our pain to another person can leave us truly powerful. Not as in "having power over," which is superficial and externally based, but as in "being secure in self," which is internal and fundamental.

Finally, there is the value of public commitment. Telling another person of our intent is crucial to carrying out difficult tasks. Research shows that when we try to stop smoking, go on a diet, or start an exercise program, we are much more apt to succeed if we tell other people about our plan. "Going public" benefits us in three ways. First, we receive a lot of support for our intended purpose. Second, we find we can handle the response of those who disagree with us or who in other ways won't support us. Third, anticipating the guilt we would feel if we didn't carry through can help energize us into action. To be completely honest with another human being, to do a Fifth Step, is a start toward our public commitment to living an honest life.

"Admitted to the God of our understanding, . . ."
In taking the first four Steps, we have become increasingly comfortable with contacting our Higher Power. Our trust in this all-loving and all-accepting Power makes the

second part of Step Five seem a natural extension of talking with ourselves.

Dan says, "Talking about it with my Higher Power seemed natural, easy. And I trusted that good would come of it. I experienced relief."

". . . to ourselves, . . ."

At this point, admitting our "shortcomings" to ourselves is perhaps the least difficult part of Step Five. We have been working at self-revelation from the beginning. We're used to it and getting pretty good at it, even though there are probably some problems we still deny. By now most of us are fairly comfortable with getting to know parts of ourselves we haven't wanted to explore. We've learned the risk is minimal because we're doing all this in our heads.

Dan says, "After I really started to think about my anger, analyze it, and see what it did to me, it wasn't so hard. Seeing it was there didn't make it any worse."

". . . and to another human being . . ."

For most of us, this is undoubtedly the most difficult requirement of Step Five. To allow another human being to see through our carefully managed presentation of ourselves to the turmoil within may seem impossible.

Jane says, "I just didn't think I could do it. I'm sixty-three and felt like a scared five-year-old. No one has ever known how I really feel about my arthritis, and I've been proud of that fact. Now I was supposed to talk about all the stuff I'd been hiding."

Jane did have to talk to another person; otherwise false pride would control her forever. She would continue to avoid the responsibility of acknowledging her whole self, the negative as well as the positive. The experience of talking with an "outsider" reduces fear and increases self-respect. Being honest with another human being will free Jane from the tension of pretending.

When we choose a person with whom to share our Fifth Step, we must choose with care. Most important, we must feel safe and comfortable with him or her. The person must be objective, have the ability to keep what we say confidential, and be able to respond to us in terms of the Twelve Steps. Since accepting feedback is an important part of this Step, we must have respect for our Fifth Step partner.

It is best to choose someone who is not a family member or close friend. With an insider, there is often too much history, too many preconceptions and personal feelings involved. Choose a nondisabled person or at least a person who does not share the same physical problem. We need someone who can be completely objective. Remember, the purpose of the Fifth Step is to admit the nature of our wrongs and the extent of our pain—we don't have to discuss changes or ask for help from our listener. It is not the job of the listener to make us feel good about ourselves. If he or she is not clearly objective, the

Fifth Step will become an exercise rather than a spiritually enriching experience.

". . . the exact nature of our wrongs."
When we find and face our pain, the tendency is to label it as powerlessness, anger, fear, despair, or something else. We identify it, but we try not to identify with it; we try not to feel it. Labeling pain is a first step, but only a first. It is one thing to say, "I am angry that I have diabetes." It is quite another to express that anger with all of the rageful emotion that our subconscious feels. If we do a Fifth Step with a listener while labeling and discussing our various feelings, it will help. But if we can express our feelings fully, detail them with examples, and show our deep vulnerability, it will help even more. This requires more energy and may even deepen our own awareness of our pain; but ultimately this kind of revelation undercuts false pride, increases humility, and promotes complete healing.

Jane says, "I knew this was going to be one of the hardest things I'd ever done, but I was determined to do it right! I really opened up to her. I showed my feelings, didn't just talk about them. And once I started, it got a life of its own and took off. I cried and laughed and beat on the arm of my chair. I was exhausted when it was over—empty and peaceful. My counselor was great. She didn't interfere with me at all. She just listened, and I knew that whatever I said was okay."

Jane was fortunate. She was able to decide, before she began, that she was going to carry the meeting through in the way she believed was in her own best interest. She would do this even though it would be very difficult and contrary to all of her past behavior. Jane was able to put aside her self-consciousness and allow her vulnerability to show. As a result, at the end of the session she felt tremendous relief.

For others, it may be a little more complicated. When they break through their denial to the exact nature and extent of their pain, they discover an overwhelming wall of shame—shame about the pain and about the chronic illness or physical challenge that caused it. That happened to Meg, who has been blind since a freak accident.

"When I started talking, I was washed with feeling—but not the feeling I was talking about. Instead I was overwhelmed with shame."

Shame supports denial. Talking with another person about the exact nature and extent of her wrongs broke Meg's denial. It exposed her shame and allowed her to work on that shame with a caring, objective, accepting person.

Step Five shows us the way out of isolation and loneliness. It teaches us that we can be our whole selves without being rejected or abandoned. It lets us see that we have the strength to face the pain within ourselves and to show it to others. It lets us see that humility can bring us into the human community.

After completing a Fifth Step, we may feel different, relieved, exalted. Or we may feel that it is just another necessary step in a lifelong process. It doesn't matter. The only important thing is carrying it out to the very best of our abilities.

We mustn't expect miracles. Insight and one cathartic experience aren't enough for real long-term change. We'll probably relapse many times. We may again become servants to our pain, which we try to deny and hide. But each time we recover, each time we recommit to honesty, each time we turn to our Higher Power for support, we make it easier for ourselves in the future. Learning to live with humility and honesty may be more difficult than learning many other things in life, but the technique is the same: practice, practice, and more practice.

After we do a Fifth Step, we find that we have two supports—our Higher Power and the memory of our Fifth Step experience. We can carry these supports with us as we slowly begin to live honest and humble lives, free of pridefulness, deceit, and grandiosity. In our new regime of honest living we will need these supports. We need them because while most people will accept and value our new beliefs and behaviors, some people—perhaps even some we love—may be uncomfortable with our change and reject us.

Many people repeat their Fifth Step from time to time. It's a good idea for two reasons. First, it reinforces a belief in our capability to be honest with ourselves, our Higher Power, and other people. Second, in repeating the experience we can always deepen it. We can move away from simple identification of our pain and toward closer identification with it. The more we know about it, the more we feel it, the more of it we will be able to release.

Step Five: Written Exercise

1. List the emotions you felt when you admitted the exact nature and extent of your pain to (a) yourself, (b) your Higher Power, and (c) another person. Make each of these lists as detailed as possible.

2. How was the feedback you received when you talked about your pain with another person? Was it helpful to you?

3. Were there ways in which you felt hurt by the feedback? If so, list them.

4. List the things you felt most uncomfortable about sharing with your Fifth Step person.

5. Were there things you felt you couldn't talk about? If so, what were they?

6. How do you feel about having completed the Fifth Step? How has it benefited you?

7. How do you feel about repeating this Step in the future?

Step Five: Imagery Exercise

Close your eyes and imagine yourself in a safe place, comfortable and relaxed. You are aware that you are going to do something difficult and that it will come out well. Enjoy the feeling.

Start thinking of all the pain you experience with your chronic illness or physical challenge. Think how it hurts you. Allow yourself to experience this.

Ask your Higher Power to join you. Explain what you are feeling and why.

Now, if you would like, ask your Fifth Step listener to join you and your Higher Power. If you feel frightened, ask your Higher Power for comfort. Take your time with this; you need to feel comfortable before continuing.

Next, imagine yourself talking about the exact nature and extent of your emotional pain. Imagine being as vulnerable as you can. Watch yourself carefully and notice how your Higher Power supports you. Again, take your time; don't rush this.

When you have said everything you want to, thank your Fifth Step person and your Higher Power for being available to you.

Open your eyes and return to your day.

Giving Up Our Pain

Step Six: Were entirely ready to have the God of our understanding remove all of our defects of character.

The traditional words of AA's Sixth and Seventh Steps may seem harsh. We don't like to feel as though we have "defects of character" or "shortcomings." But what these words really mean is that we are human—we have attitudes and behaviors that lead us to live with emotional pain. Our job is to work with the Steps so that our "defects," "shortcomings," and self-destructive attitudes and behaviors will be replaced by emotional strength, integrity, and faith.

Step Six asks again for deep introspection. We get a chance to look at the effect that unconscious motivation has on our lives. First, Step Six questions our readiness to change. Are we entirely, absolutely ready to give up the way we have learned to be, the way we are? Are we ready to live without the emotional pain attached to our chronic illness or disability? Are we ready to give up the behaviors that go with that pain? Second, this Step questions our commitment to trusting and having faith in our Higher Power. Do we believe that our Higher Power cares enough, or is strong enough, to help us? If we are ready to give up our pain and our dysfunctional behaviors, and if we believe in our relationship with our Higher Power, Step Six assures us of spiritual growth.

"Were entirely ready . . ."
When asked if we are ready to live without emotional pain and the destructive behavior that goes with it, our immediate response is, "Of course. If there were a choice, who would want to continue this way?" The reality is that we have.

Early in our chronic illness or disability we took on emotional pain and destructive behaviors as the best response to the situation. They were the least threatening of all possible reactions. This seems hard to believe; but remember, for the most part we learn and maintain feelings and actions that help us survive. They may be poor choices, but at the time of crisis they seem like the least of the evils. We make a conscious decision to define, feel, and behave in a certain way, and those reactions become ingrained and habitual. We actually become comfortable with our pain—it is a known entity, and we are practiced in handling it. We choose to stay with the predictability of our current way of being.

In many ways our pain protected and helped us. Shock and denial protect us from the mind-shattering pain of initial discovery or diagnosis. Feelings of powerlessness are realistic responses to a situation beyond our control. Fear, anxiety, depression, and grief all can act as tools of power. We may gain a sense of control as we use them to manipulate the feelings and behavior of other people. Grief and powerlessness can get us support. Anger, rage, blaming, and isolation may keep others at a "safe" distance. Pain can keep our attention on ourselves so we don't have to take risks with others. And pain can protect us from having to accept ourselves and get on with life and personal growth. Our pain helps us to feel as though we are in some way controlling and managing our lives. It is familiar and predictable; we know how it works.

In practicing the Sixth Step, keep in mind we are dealing with our irrational, subconscious mind rather than our rational consciousness. Our subconscious mind tries to maintain the status quo. It fights hard against any decision our conscious mind makes toward change. This is understandable. We face several powerful threats if we choose to accept our whole selves and begin to live without pain.

First, there is the issue of predictability and security.

We may not like how we feel and act, but we are familiar with it—there are no surprises. Second, and closely related, is our fear of the unknown and of taking risks. Third, there is the question of the void. If we let go of our present emotions, what will we put in their place? For many depressed people, the idea of being outgoing and active is so frightening that they feel physically ill when they think about it. Those filled with rage and anger often say, "If I imagine that the anger is gone, there's this empty place in me." Or, "If I'm not angry, then what's going to push me?"

Finally, there is the fear of facing what our pain is trying to hide. The truth is that many of us are afraid of being what we are—chronically ill or physically challenged people. This is our life, our only life; we are going to live it within constraints that most people don't experience and can't understand.

Spiritual growth, the very heart of the Twelve Step program, takes place through our subconscious. Our conscious mind has done what it can. It has lectured us, threatened us, bargained with us, pleaded with us to let go of our pain and change our ways. None of that has worked. Now we need to let the Twelve Steps take over. We need to surround ourselves with the spiritual resources that will work within our subconscious mind, to nurture us, to hear us, to melt away the threat. With the Sixth Step we recommit ourselves to the care of a Power greater than ourselves. Our faith in this Power and our trust that it can remove our pain and change our lives is our foundation of strength and hope.

*". . . to have the God of our understanding remove all of our de-
fects of character."*

Step Six doesn't require that we take charge of removing
our self-destructive behaviors and our pain. It centers on
the fact that we can't do it by ourselves. In AA it's often
said, "You alone can do it, but you can't do it alone." We
don't need to be active; we just need to be ready. We simply allow ourselves a state of mind, a state of being, that is
willing to let go. We must be willing to surrender our pain
to our Higher Power, be willing to finally live without it.
Our ability to do this is a measure of our humility. As in
Step Three, we must give over our will and our ego. It is
the support of the spiritual resources that surround us
which can remove our pain, not the will of our conscious
mind.

Some people come easily to the point where they feel
entirely ready to have their pain removed; some think
they are ready but find their will still in control, refusing
to let go. Most of us move very slowly in this Step. To
help, some of us use the Serenity Prayer:

God, grant me the serenity
To accept the things I cannot change,
The courage to change the things I can,
And the wisdom to know the difference.

Some of us create our own version of this traditional
prayer. Others may have other affirmations, mantras, or
meditations that they find meaningful and helpful.
Slowly and with much effort we move toward the place
where we can believe in life without our pain. Slowly we

deepen the humility that will make that life possible. Slowly we move on toward the Seventh Step.

Step Seven: Humbly asked God to remove our shortcomings.

To successfully work the Seventh Step, we must have self-respect, we must be humble, and we must exercise faith. These three elements come together in a process that works to remove emotional pain. To honestly ask our Higher Power to help us, we must first respect ourselves enough to believe that we deserve to live without pain. We must believe in our personal value and integrity. As we do this, we say, "I'm looking for a better way; I'm worth struggling for." Second, we must be able to accept ourselves and our place without denial or grandiosity. We must be humble if we are to sincerely ask for help and sincerely receive it. Third, we must have faith. Exercising faith gives us the energy that makes the process work. We may have self-respect and be humble, but without the energy of faith, we cannot have a relationship with a Higher Power, and our pain cannot be removed.

"Humbly asked God . . ."
In Step Seven we don't request, plead, insist, or bargain. We "humbly ask" our Higher Power to remove our pain. To be humble is the requirement. Humility is a natural consequence of the Twelve Step program, and only through humility can we live it. Step One asks us to

understand humility by accepting our powerlessness. Step Two requires that we acknowledge a Power outside of and greater than ourselves. Step Three deepens our humility by suggesting that we turn over our life and will to this Power in the belief that it, better than we, can lead us to spiritual growth and fulfillment. Steps Four and Five increase both our humility and self-respect as we identify, accept, and acknowledge to another person the extent of our shortcomings. Finally, in Steps Six and Seven our humility allows us to ask for the active intervention of our Higher Power.

". . . to remove our shortcomings."
We need to put ourselves in a frame of mind in which our shortcomings can be removed. We have to be willing to let go of our self-destructive feelings and be available to our Higher Power. So, how do we do this?

Delores, who is being treated for a melanoma (a malignant tumor) on her back, says, "All I say is help, help. I don't ask for anything."

Cathy just had an ileostomy (a permanent removal of her lower bowel) to relieve her life-threatening colitis. She doesn't ask for help; she just admits her pain, over and over: "I am so frightened; I am so frightened."

When we talk with our Higher Power, the dialogue will be more successful if we remember that the kind of request that begins "I want to _____ [be less angry, feel more secure]" doesn't work. This way of framing our request asks our Higher Power to support our will. The whole point of Step Seven is to acknowledge that our will hasn't worked, that we need to look to the will of a Power greater than ourselves to relieve us.

We have to be able to recognize the things we want our Higher Power to remove. Because our pain and our behavior are so habitual, it's often hard to recognize them when they occur. Some people find it helpful to imagine a separate part of themselves that stands outside to observe. The job of this observer is not to be judgmental or critical but to be objective. When the observer notices a negative feeling or a behavior that represents this feeling, it reminds us to call for help from a Higher Power.

Another way to work with Step Seven is to try new behaviors, to ask our Higher Power to suggest ways to break out of old patterns.

Rhoda says her husband gets impatient when he gets tied into her dialysis routine. "Sometimes he has to rearrange business meetings to take me to an appointment when, for some reason, I can't drive myself or there's some other kind of problem. I used to always feel guilty, hurt, and angry, but I wouldn't say anything. I would just go out of my way to try to make it up to him.

"Then, one day, when this situation came up and I got the old feelings, I stopped and asked my Higher Power to tell me how this could change. Lo and behold, I got the idea to make an arrangement with my neighbor, Rosalie. If I could count on her to take me to dialysis when I couldn't get there by myself, she could count on me for emergency baby-sitting. Then I told my husband about how I felt and what I'd worked out with

Rosalie. He felt guilty at first, but we talked about that too, so now it's a lot better. I don't know why I didn't think of this sooner—my Higher Power has great ideas, but I was so busy feeling miserable I couldn't hear them."

In the course of living with our disability or illness, we have learned patterns of behavior that have become deeply ingrained habits. Even though many of them are unhealthy and may increase our pain, they are behaviors we know, and it will take much hard and committed work for us to allow our Higher Power to remove them. We can go slowly, remembering the strength of "One day at a time," or "Patience is always an alternative." Some of our steps will be baby steps. We will lose a little fear in one situation and be relieved of a little anger in another. We can acknowledge the change, be grateful for it, and look forward to more. Some of us may experience giant steps. We may wake up on the other side of depression or find ourselves going to bed at night with surplus energy. We may never lose all of our negative feelings, but we can learn to use the "hangers on" in positive ways. Instead of letting feelings of isolation fill us with the pain of loneliness, we can use them to indicate a need to separate from others and rest. Powerlessness can increase our awareness of our relationship with our Higher Power. We can use anger as constructive energy, rather than in ways that hurt ourselves or others. And we can use fear as an impetus to search for knowledge about whatever it is we're afraid of.

For the Seventh Step to work, it doesn't matter how we perceive our Higher Power. It's only necessary that we have self-respect, be humble, and have faith that our Power can help us.

Meg's God is a traditional one. She prays: "Please see my pain and help me to understand Your Will for me. My life is in Your hands."

Dan's Higher Power is the Twelve Step program. He asks: "Help me live by your principles. Help me let go of my pain and find a better way."

Jane, whose Higher Power is a White Light that comes from within, never really asks for help. "I just decided to concentrate on living the program as I understood it. My fears about my future have evaporated. Today seems more important than tomorrow. And rarely, rarely, do I get angry or discouraged anymore. There's no reason to. I am who I am and that's good.

Steps Six and Seven: Written Exercise

1. As you begin to work Step Six, ask yourself how ready you are on a scale of one to ten to have your Higher Power remove your shortcomings.
2. Of the eight major kinds of emotional pain described in Step Four's inventory (powerlessness; fear and anxiety; isolation; anger and rage; ambiguity and blame; jealousy; grief; and exhaustion), which play the biggest role in your life?
3. Which destructive feelings have been most useful to you? Describe how they've helped.

4. Which of them will be most difficult to let go? Why?

5. Which will be the easiest to release?

6. Which of them do you think have the potential of acting as positives instead of negatives? How will this work for you?

7. How can your subconscious mind control your emotional pain?

8. Why does humility play such an important role in working Steps Six and Seven?

9. What is your most effective way of communicating with your Higher Power?

Steps Six and Seven: Imagery Exercise

Imagine yourself in a safe place. You are relaxed and comfortable. Your Higher Power is with you.

Imagine a painful feeling. Allow an image that represents that feeling to come into your mind. Take time. Let your subconscious mind give you whatever it will. When you can see or sense the presence of your negative feeling, take it in your hands. Take time to experience how it feels to hold it.

Allow your Higher Power to take the painful image from you. Remain completely willing to let go. As it is taken from you, notice what happens to the image. Notice also how it feels to give away your pain. Stay with that feeling. If you are uncomfortable, ask your Higher Power for support; if you are relieved, give thanks.

Open your eyes. Repeat this exercise as often as you wish, applying it to different painful feelings.

CHAPTER ELEVEN

Making Amends

Step Eight: Made a list of all persons we had harmed, and became willing to make amends to them all.

"Impossible," "No way!" "How would I dare?" These are all common responses to what Step Eight asks of us. "There are just too many people. My friends, my family, doctors, nurses, lab techs, and receptionists—there's no end to it." Seemingly there *is* no end. Once we truly accept how we have behaved, many of us are overwhelmed by the enormity of what working Step Eight would mean.

Also, we are frightened by the new pain we may face. "Just the thought of looking at all that makes me so guilty, I can hardly stand it. Can't I just forget the past and get on with what I am doing with myself now?" The answer is no. In the first place, we can't forget the past; we can only fire up our denial to suppress it. The best we can do is use our emotional energy to push it into our sub-conscious, where it will continue to fester. This is the way we have done things in the past, and we know that hasn't worked. It's denial, it's dishonest, and it's self-destructive.

When we get past our immediate rejection of the idea of making amends, we can slow down and think about it. The Twelve Steps have given us the tools to atone for our past. We know what it means to be honest; we have faith that our Higher Power is with us and will care for us; we have an increased sense of self-respect; and we have the experience of the Fifth Step to carry with us. All we need to do is allow ourselves to spend whatever time we need nurturing ourselves, communicating with our Higher Power, and just getting used to the idea.

When we are faced with an enormous problem, it always helps to break it down into smaller pieces. First, we'll look at our feelings about what we have to do and then clarify what making amends actually means.

Most of us are afraid of the feelings we will have when we face the people we've harmed and acknowledge how we have hurt them. We may be afraid we will look foolish. We may be afraid we'll feel guilt, regret, remorse, or shame. Guilt and regret are healthy responses in this situation. Guilt, which comes when our behavior conflicts with our personal values, is certainly appropriate. Regret, which means to look back on an event with sorrow or to be distressed because of it, makes good sense too. But remorse (self-accusatory regret) and shame (the viewing of ourselves as worthless) are unhealthy responses. We need to carefully search our reaction and decide which of these emotions we are feeling. Then we need to turn to our Higher Power to help us deal with false pride, remorse, and shame.

When we think of making amends, most of us think of apologizing—and that's not it. Amends are not apologies. Apologies mean saying we're sorry; amends mean changing behavior. Many times in our anger we lash out at a friend or loved one. Then we apologize. Then we become angry and lash out again. Then we apologize. And on and on. Nothing changes. Amends may include an apology but are also much more. When we make amends, we acknowledge what we have done, accept full responsibility for it, and make a commitment never to repeat the harmful action. These are true amends. It's very hard, but it's not impossible. And it's essential for spiritual wellness.

After working the first seven Steps, we have come to realize that we have to let go of the past and put our emotional energy into living in the present. Amends are important because we cannot build a good present when our hurtful past lies hidden in our subconscious. It eats up our energy and keeps us bound to old feelings that may interfere with every day of our lives. The only way to break this pattern is to let go of our denial about the past. We can admit that in our pain we have hurt ourselves and others. We can make our amends. Then we can learn to be honest in the present, to respect ourselves, and to treat others with honesty and respect as well. The Eighth Step prepares the way for that to happen.

"Made a list of all persons we had harmed, . . ."
This list starts with our own name. It's imperative that we make amends to ourselves first; otherwise, we can't sincerely or effectively make amends to others. It's like love and respect—we have to give it to ourselves before we can pass it on.

Our commitment to living by the Twelve Step program is the foundation for making amends to ourselves. We are committed to changing our thoughts, beliefs, and behavior. Until now, we have abused ourselves. We have spent hours, days, months, perhaps years, abusing our minds with the stress of negative emotions. We have exchanged days and nights of our lives for emotional pain we cannot manage. We have also abused our relationships with others. We have lost lots of time; we have lost friends, loved ones, and intimacy. Working the Steps and making amends to ourselves allows us time to grieve for our losses and to let our Higher Power help us deal with this grief.

". . . and became willing to make amends to them all."
When we have made amends to ourselves, we can begin the process of making amends to others. On our list we put anyone and everyone we can think of whom we have harmed. It can include spouses, children, parents, lovers, friends, colleagues, and acquaintances. Sometimes we may have been deliberately hurtful. Sometimes we were blind to the injury we caused.

Growing Stronger

Step Nine: Made direct amends to such people wherever possible, except when to do so would injure them or others.

Beginning to take the Ninth Step is like standing on the threshold of a new life. We are learning to live with humility and honesty in the present; but if this new life is to have real integrity, we must put our past life in order. We want to build our house on firm ground, not quicksand. Step Eight has led us to this point: We know what we need to do; now we have to do it. We have acknowledged to ourselves the ways in which we have hurt others. Now we must acknowledge that hurt to each of our victims.

Working the Ninth Step not only helps us to resolve our past, but it also strengthens the special traits that help our spirit grow. It takes courage to stand face-to-face with someone we have truly harmed and say, "I know that I hurt you, I am responsible for doing it, I deeply regret it, and I pledge to you that I won't ever do it again." It takes insight, thoughtfulness, and wisdom to choose the amends that will be most beneficial to each individual we have harmed. It takes patience, reflection, and planning to find the most appropriate time and method to carry out our amends. It takes deep understanding of our need to resolve the past in order to free ourselves of the future. Finally, it takes vigilance to protect ourselves against the denial that could cause us to avoid making particular amends.

Making amends is an ongoing process of resolving our emotional conflicts. It is not something we can do quickly and get over with. Carrying them out in a thoughtful, thorough way becomes a part of life as we work the Twelve Steps. It continually deepens our humility. As our spirituality grows, we may recognize more situations in which our pain has hurt others and know that the only way to erase that hurt for both the other person and ourselves is to make amends.

Carrying out Step Nine can bring great benefits. Each time we make amends, we lose guilt and resentment and gain self-respect, courage, confidence, and self-esteem. This can happen no matter how the other person responds. When the person accepts our amends and supports our efforts, our spirit is enriched. If it goes badly, if the other person is angry, disrespectful, and lashes out at us, we still know that we have taken responsibility for our actions, so we grow from that too. To endear ourselves to the people we have harmed is not the object; the object is to live one day at a time with self-respect and integrity.

"Made direct amends to such people wherever possible, . . ." Making direct amends means to take candid, straightforward action. What form that direct action takes will depend on the availability of the person involved. If possible, we should meet the person face-to-face. This is the most intimate, and therefore the most effective, way of presenting amends. It is appropriate to telephone first, explaining that we would like a meeting. We don't have to give any special reason; in fact, it's preferable not to get bogged down in an explanation at this point.

Most people find it harder to go to enemies than to friends or loved ones. For some, the closer the relationship with the harmed person, the more difficult the amends. Some of us like to make our most difficult amends first, "to get them over with"; some start out with less-threatening amends to "practice on the easier ones." If we reflect quietly, ask for the advice of our Higher

Power, and simply wait for a response, we will know who our first contact should be.

In a few cases, the person we have harmed may be unaware of what we have done. He or she doesn't know we suffer guilt and regret, so it's very easy to avoid these amends. "What difference does it make?" we think to ourselves. "She doesn't know, so why should I upset things?" The fact that she may not be aware of what we have done is irrelevant. It's our awareness of wrongdoing that matters; it's our subconscious that must carry the pain until we make amends. When we have the courage to approach these people, we show the depth of our commitment to the Twelve Steps and our intention to live an honest and humble life. The visit may be awkward and have consequences we don't like, but to avoid it is to allow old patterns of denial and rationalization to take over. To carry it through enriches our spirit.

We will probably need to make amends to some people that we won't be able to meet face-to-face. They may live far away or be unavailable for some other reason. These amends can be made by telephone or through letters. Phoning is the more direct way, because we have to deal with the other person's immediate response. It's often useful to follow up our call with a letter. Avoiding the telephone and making amends by mail alone is attractive because it's easier and less threatening, but it's a one-sided communication. By itself, letter writing makes the least effective amends, and it sidesteps our responsibility.

It's just as important to make amends to people we can't contact at all because they have died or we have lost touch with them. There are several ways to do this. We can have conversations with them, either in our imagination or, more effectively, by pretending we are with them. We visualize them sitting with us and make our amends, speaking out loud to them. This is our way of putting the relationship to rest and releasing ourselves at the same time. Another method is to write a long, detailed letter to the person, even though it will never be mailed. Finally, we can make our amends to someone who has died or disappeared by searching out and assisting a relative or other individual important to the person we harmed. We can explain our motivation, or not, whichever seems appropriate.

Making Your First Amends

Guidelines can help when we plan to make amends.

1. Plan. Be thorough in your preparation. Be sure of what you want to say. Spend as much time as you need with your Higher Power, asking advice and listening to the response. Each kind of amends will be different, based on the situation, so plan carefully each time.

2. Don't go into it with expectations about how the other person will respond. Simply be respectful and understand that you must accept whatever happens. You don't have control over the outcome, only over your part in the process.

3. Ask permission first and be willing to accept the other's response. Some victims may choose not to

hear your amends, and that's their right. Others may choose not to accept it, and you have to respect this too. We must not gain our peace of mind by being disrespectful.

4. Be careful to put the responsibility for what happened on your own shoulders. Speak only of your part in the hurtful situation; don't comment on behavior of the other. If you have remaining resentment or anger, the amends aren't valid.

5. Keep it simple and straightforward.

6. Whatever the other's response, remain calm, humble, and without anger or resentment.

7. Be willing to forgive yourself and the other person, and when the amends have been made, release your pain to your Higher Power.

Jane, who has rheumatoid arthritis, and Dan, who has heart disease, both had a great deal of anxiety as they began to work Step Nine. Jane chose to approach a friend, while Dan made his first amends to one of his original doctors, who had died.

Jane: "I met with her and told her I knew how my rejection of her offers of help and friendship had hurt her. I was very explicit about the specific pain that I was suffering that made me act the way I did. I asked for her forgiveness but told her that whether or not she could forgive me, I wanted her to know how deeply I regretted that I had locked her out of my life. She didn't exactly fall into my arms, but we are working out a new relationship. Her trust is growing. We're still friends."

Dan: "I wanted to make amends to my first doctor. He tried hard to help me, but I was so mad at that point, and I took most of it out on him. When he died, I felt guilty but put it out of my mind. Every time I thought of him, I pushed the thought away. So for the Ninth Step I wrote him a letter. I told him how angry I was at that time, how I knew that I'd been awful to him, and that I really felt sorry about it now. I know how hard he tried to help me; he was a good person and a good doctor. And I told him I was doing great now. I actually cried when I wrote it. Then I wrote a letter to his wife and told her how important her husband had been to me, that he had been a fine man. It's okay to think about him now—I feel much better."

". . . except when to do so would injure them or others."
There is an exception to making direct amends. If we think we might harm someone by making full amends to them, or that our disclosures might hurt a third person, we need to be very careful about how we proceed. First, we must be sure that we are not rationalizing our avoidance, that our concern is genuine. Prayer or meditation will help, and consultation with an objective outsider is a good reality check. If we decide that partial amends are necessary to avoid giving the other person more pain, it's appropriate to set limits on what we say. These kinds of amends will protect the victim and still give us full benefit. While we make partial amends verbally, we silently make full amends—a commitment to a changed behavior.

Steps Eight and Nine: Written Exercise

1. Explain how making amends will help you release the past. Why is this important?
2. What are your major fears about making amends? How can you overcome them?
3. What is the difference between amends and an apology?
4. List three people to whom you need to make amends and explain why.
5. Write out your amends to yourself.
6. After making amends to yourself, what are the most important amends you can make?
7. Who will it be the most difficult to make amends to? Why?
8. Are there people to whom you feel it would not be appropriate to make full amends? Who? Why?
9. How can your Higher Power help you make amends?

Steps Eight and Nine: Imagery Exercise

Imagine you are making a list of people to whom you need to make amends. The list doesn't have to be absolutely complete; you can repeat this exercise as often as necessary.

Choose someone on the list and carefully plan your amends. Use your spiritual resources for support.

Imagine being with the person to whom you will make amends. Imagine the scene in as much detail as possible.

Make your amends. When you are finished, thank the person you harmed for hearing your amends.

Take time to experience the feeling of having completed your amends. Then return to your day, knowing that this exercise will help you when the time comes to make amends in real life.

CHAPTER TWELVE

Spiritual Awakening

Step Ten: Continued to take personal inventory and when we were wrong promptly admitted it.

In working Steps One through Nine we have learned to change our way of being. We have built a new spiritual base; we have both identified and identified *with* our pain. We have learned how to relieve the negative feelings that have controlled us and have come to terms with our past. Our lives are now different, better. We have given up our attempts to control the outcome. We have learned to take responsibility only for the process and to trust that the process will take us where we need to go. We have a new will for loving. Most of us experience a sense of peace, of comfort, of being in place. We are on the other side of Step Nine, and the question is, how do we prevent relapse and continue our growth?

Jane explains how she feels: "Things are so different; I am so different. Sometimes I get scared I'll lose it."

Rhoda says: "I'm used to living by the program now. It's habit. I'm afraid that I'm not paying attention to it the way I should. I sure don't want to fall back to the way I was before."

Steps Ten through Twelve show us how to deal with what Jane and Rhoda are afraid of. In Step Ten, we learn a method to maintain our new life pattern. Step Eleven helps us deepen our understanding and commitment. Step Twelve shows us how to continue our growth by reaching beyond our own lives. These last three Steps ask for our commitment to continue work, and that means a commitment to our growing spiritual strength and wellness. When we accept the program as a lifelong process, the need to immediately reach our goal diminishes, and we relax into our new self.

"Continued to take personal inventory . . ."
It takes at least six months to integrate new thinking patterns or behavior into our lives. Even after that, we have periods of relapse. A recovering smoker will have an urge for a cigarette four, or even twenty-four years, after he or she has stopped smoking. Stress, difficult times, or life crises can bring about old behavior. It seems that when things get tough, our oldest, most ingrained, and most familiar, gut-level feelings resurface and take over. Most of us understand this and watch out. We should also be vigilant at ordinary times—when we have the flu or a cold, when we're tired, when we haven't been eating well, when we're just not quite "on." At these times, too, we're vulnerable to fall back into our "favorite" emotional pains.

We need to keep the program at the front of our consciousness so we can act on it rather than react to negative circumstances. We need to develop small daily rituals that keep us constantly aware of our new pattern of living. Otherwise, we can slip, by omission, back into our old self-destructive ways.

Staying on Top

There are three techniques for maintaining consciousness of the program.

Spot-check inventory. Several times a day we stop and quickly review our feelings and behavior. In this way, when we slip, we make prompt repairs. Perhaps we need to refer back to the Third Step, or the Fourth, or to make immediate amends. We do whatever seems appropriate, and we do it promptly. We can also use a spot-check when a question or dilemma arises for which we don't have an easy answer. Then we take time to go back over what we have learned and respond accordingly. The more we do this, the less we will find ourselves "losing it" to our old thoughts and actions.

Daily inventory. The daily inventory serves a different purpose. Although this inventory has to be done daily, it doesn't have to be long, or complicated, or time-consuming. We can do it as we are brushing our teeth, getting ready for bed, or perhaps just before we go to sleep. Doing this inventory as a ritual can remind us that the Twelve Steps is a program we live one day at a time. It keeps us focused on the present and helps us give up anxiety about either the past or the future. We ask ourselves: Did I feel an old familiar pain today? If so, what did I do about it? Could I have handled it differently or better? Do I need to make amends? If I do, when and how will I do it? Did I slip back into controlling, managing, or manipulating others? Did I truly surrender the outcome? The daily practice of this inventory helps us to maintain honesty and humility, and leads to continuing spiritual growth.

Long-term inventory. This inventory is done a few times a year. We set aside enough time for a comprehensive look at how we have been doing. We look at our progress from a long-term perspective, getting a clear picture of our gains and where we need to focus our work in the future. Many of us like to use this time to celebrate our progress—and be thankful.

". . . and when we were wrong promptly admitted it."
We are going to relapse—some of us more than others. As we work the Twelve Steps, we have to accept relapse as a part of our new life. Like a former smoker who has a cigarette, we can relapse into pain and the behavior that goes with it. It's inevitable. The Tenth Step is designed to help us realize that relapse is not the end of the world.

When we do a spot-check and a daily inventory, we can catch relapses quickly and promptly repair them. Promptness is crucial. If we allow ourselves to drop back into our old ways, we are apt to feel guilty or ashamed over our relapse. When we are prompt in making our repairs, feelings of guilt and shame can't drive us into a pit of self-hatred. We won't have to use denial, rationalization, and grandiosity to cover our disgust. These spirit destroyers don't have a chance to get rooted, so they can't undercut our spiritual healing. Remember, when we fall back to our old ways, we haven't lost all that we've gained. We just have to get back to doing the things that keep us emotionally healthy.

The Tenth Step is program maintenance. Here we recognize that we can relapse into emotional pain. We admit that we have a problem with old feelings and behaviors, and promptly make repairs. It is a point from which we can go back and recommit to what we already know and move forward to deepening and expanding our spirit.

Step Ten: Written Exercise

1. When we do the spot-check and daily inventories, what emotional pains seem to keep reappearing?
2. Which of them seem to have disappeared?
3. What is the value of spot-check inventories?
4. What is the value of daily inventories?
5. What is the value of long-term inventories?
6. What does the phrase "The Tenth Step is the maintenance Step" mean to you?
7. Why does Step Ten help us toward spiritual growth one day at a time?

Step Ten: Imagery Exercise

Imagine yourself driving, taking a walk, washing dishes, exercising, taking a bath or shower, any ordinary activity—something you do alone every day. Just be there with yourself.

Do a spot-check inventory. Look back at how your day has been and see how you are doing.

Imagine that you remember feeling an old, familiar pain or behaving in a way that reflects a negative emotion. Decide what you need to do to repair the situation and release yourself from it. Take your time; do a complete job of repair.

Re-enter your day, keeping in mind the importance of the Tenth Step message.

CHAPTER THIRTEEN

Gaining Peace

Step Eleven: Sought through prayer and meditation to improve our conscious contact with the God of our understanding, praying only for knowledge of God's will for us and the power to carry that out.

The purpose of Step Eleven is to reaffirm for us, each day, the first three Steps of the program. To admit our powerlessness, to recognize a healing Power outside of ourselves, and to turn our will and our lives over to the support of our spiritual resources have given us the strength to turn our lives around. Now we have to keep it that way. This Step is our chance to develop an ever-deepening awareness of our Higher Power and the peace that comes with that relationship. It is a daily recommitment to our spirituality.

Step Eleven works in tandem with Step Ten. As we carry out our spot-check and daily inventories, we use conscious contact with our Higher Power to help and sustain us. And, like the inventories of Step Ten, daily meditation or prayer keeps the program in our consciousness and keeps it growing. We may feel a letdown when we have passed through the initial excitement and dedication to our new way of life—the Eleventh Step helps us deal with that. It's like love. First there is the romantic attraction, thrilling in its newness and possibility. Eventually this passes, and we are ready to begin to learn to love deeply, to become completely involved and intimate with our loved one, in good times and in bad. Living within the belief system of the Twelve Steps is the process of love, love for the very deepest and most important part of ourselves: our spiritual core.

"Sought through prayer and meditation to improve our conscious contact with the God of our understanding, . . ."

Three previous Steps have called for us to make "conscious contact" with our Higher Power. Step Three asked us to turn over our will and our lives. Step Five asked us to admit our emotional pain, and Step Seven asked to have our pain removed. All these Steps involved direct, conscious communications with spiritual resources greater than ourselves. Now Step Eleven seeks to improve that communication.

The method we choose to improve our "conscious contact" will differ, depending on our beliefs. Some of us will pray; some will meditate. It absolutely does not matter which form we use. If we are faithful in practicing whichever technique is comfortable for us and are humble and sincere, our relationship with our Higher Power can become stronger.

For much of the world, the traditional way to contact a Higher Power is through prayer. Praying involves asking for what we want and asking for guidance. Most of us start out learning prayers that ask for something important to us: "God bless Mommy, Daddy, Puff, and Spot." "Have Santa Claus bring me a new doll." "Please don't let Grandma die." It's only later, as we move from the self-centeredness of childhood and become mature adults, that we learn to say, "Thy will be done." Now as we work this Step we must keep in mind that our request for guidance must always supersede "I want," no matter how important the "I want" is.

Meg, who is blind, says, "I have a special time set aside every morning after I wake up, but I'm still in bed. No one knows I'm awake when I spend a few minutes praying. I say 'The Serenity Prayer' and the 'Our Father.' Sometimes I pray for guidance about something in my life that I am dealing with; then I'm quiet and wait to see what I hear. I pray at other times during the day too, and sometimes I just have conversations with God about something or other, but I never miss those morning prayers."

Those of us who were not raised in, or have moved away from, traditional religion often use a different channel through which to communicate with our Higher Power. We may follow the Eastern practice of meditation. Meditation helps us learn to quiet our minds and rid us of the daily "noise" that fills our consciousness. When we remove the barriers of conscious thought, our Higher Power enters our minds, and in the stillness we can receive the guidance we ask for.

Jane tells us how she practices meditation:

I sit quietly and empty my mind of whatever confusion is there. I concentrate on relaxing my body too. Then I take a few deep breaths and let my White Light fill my mind. I just sit and look at it—and I always have healing thoughts come to me.

Dan's Higher Power is the program itself. This is how he explains his meditation:

"I don't like to call it meditating, but my friends tell me that's what I'm doing. What I do is be quiet, someplace by myself, and just think about the program, what it says and what it means to me. Nothing else, no particular problem, just the program. The thing that happens is that I always seem to have a part of it come to mind that turns out to be helpful in something that I'm dealing with in my life at that point. I've come to rely on it."

". . . praying only for knowledge of God's will for us and the power to carry that out."

Seeking guidance toward spiritual wellness is hard and may continue to cause us problems. It's so easy to fall back into rigidly trying to manage our lives and assuming that our Higher Power should support our will. Again and again we need to give up our attempts to control, to accept our powerlessness, to seek guidance—it's the only way to the spiritual health we're looking for. Controlling keeps us focused outward, watching ourselves managing others. Step Eleven helps us increase our inward focus, and that focus becomes clearer through our Higher Power. It encourages our spirit to take root in the fertile soil of that internal relationship.

Spiritual growth can result from the awareness that our Higher Power's guidance should direct our lives, not our own willfulness. We can remember that our basic tasks are to be open-minded about reality and to be willing to change.

Anita, who lives with severe chronic asthma says, "I've struggled and struggled with this 'will' business. I've come to think that maybe accepting my Higher Power's 'will' for me just means that I should accept reality as it is, without denial and without trying to control everything."

One side of Joe's face droops as a result of the stroke he suffered five years ago, but the other side lifts in a smile. He says, "I think the evidence that my prayers for guidance are answered shows up when I have opportunities to act in the old way and instead choose the new one. I figured that when I've done this enough times, the new way will become the old way, the old old way will be gone, and I will have received guidance."

Anita and Joe describe the practical essence of Step Eleven. We can find the guidance of our Higher Power as we accept reality, without denial, and apply the Twelve Step program. In this way, we can learn to cope with the stress of day-to-day living without painful emotions turning it into dis-stress. Acceptance of our reality can give us a sense of peace, even when that reality contains lots of difficult and active living. It's like Yoga exercises. We stretch and work our body tremendously while focusing our minds on our quiet spiritual core. Although life may be very strenuous on the outside, it's very serene within.

Step Eleven: Written Exercise

1. What does prayer mean to you?
2. What does meditation mean to you?
3. What (prayer or meditation) is the more comfortable method for you to use in your "conscious contact" with whatever spiritual resources surround you? Explain why.
4. What emotional roadblocks interfere with your deepening contact with your Higher Power? What do you need to do to get past them?
5. List three situations in which prayer or meditation has resulted in the guidance you asked for.

Step Eleven: Imagery Exercise

Imagine yourself sitting alone in a quiet, safe place. Relax and become comfortable. See yourself as ready to make "conscious contact" with your Higher Power.

Imagine yourself carrying out Step Eleven, praying or meditating. Experience the feeling. Take your time with this; imagine your complete prayer or meditation.

When you have finished your prayer or meditation, thank your Higher Power for giving you guidance.

Come back to your day, remembering that whenever you need guidance about a concern, or simply feel the desire for contact, your own chosen spiritual resources are always available to you.

Sharing Newfound Peace

Step Twelve: Having had a spiritual awakening as the result of these steps, we tried to carry this message to others with chronic illness or disability, and to practice these principles in all our affairs.

When we started the Twelve Steps, our goal was spiritual health despite our physical conditions. Now we have been introduced to the entire program—one Step at a time. We have carried out each Step to the best of our ability and are willing to commit ourselves to reworking them whenever necessary. Our lives have changed. Today our real selves are the selves we show the world; we no longer hide them under layers of emotional pain. Our behavior has changed too. We have better friendships and family life as we relate to others with honesty and humility. Our spirits are now rooted, growing strong and healthy. We know what it is to have moments of peace, serenity, and joy.

"Having had a spiritual awakening as the result of these steps, . . ."
Most of us are not exactly sure how our spiritual awakening has come about. It may have started somewhere back in the first Steps and sort of happened along the way. It's come from an accumulation of mini-miracles and spiritual experiences that have resulted in joyful acceptance of our powerlessness, and in faith that our Higher Power will truly care for us always. We know that our spiritual awakening can continue until we die.

Meg has found a way to live with her Christian God and find peace. Jane has found a "path with heart," a way to live in harmony with the universe.

Our spiritual awakenings have taken different forms, but we have found similar gifts. We have a new basis for living, knowing we aren't alone. We no longer need to be afraid of reality, neither the reality of who we are nor what our lives are like. And we have confidence in our strength to continue this new way of being.

Our spiritual awakening has been accompanied by a change in values. Perhaps we used to value isolation because it separated us from others and allowed us to hide our pain. Now we value intimacy and connection with the world around us. Perhaps we used to value our denial because it supported our false reality. Now we value clarity and openness in our relationships with others and with ourselves. Perhaps we used to value our anger as self-protection. Now we use its power as helpful energy for positive growth. Perhaps we used to value our powerlessness as a tool to manipulate others. Now we value it because it connects us to our Higher Power and leads to serenity.

". . . we tried to carry this message to others with chronic illness or disability, and to practice these principles in all our affairs."

We know how the program works. We have had our baptism of fire as we experienced it for ourselves; now we need to carry its message beyond our own lives. Reaching out to others continues our growth; it gives us increasing knowledge, new insights, intimacy, and the miracle of seeing other people change. It's not hard to do. We don't need any special expertise, only humility and compassion. We pass on what we have learned by presenting ourselves and telling of our struggle. Our story gives others a model for behavior and the gift of hope. As we tell it, we receive a gift too. We see our old ways in people just beginning the program, and we see how far we have come. We watch others who have gone before us and see how much more we can hope to accomplish.

One of the most effective ways to carry our message is to participate in groups of other chronically ill or disabled people. (See appendix E.) Groups provide support, understanding, and empathy from those whose life experiences are much like our own—and who share the emotional pain we know so well. In groups we can trust that others will accept us as we are. As we allow others to know us, we are practicing and reaping the rewards of honesty. We get reality checks when we talk about our lives and people respond, reinforcing the beliefs of the Twelve Steps and helping us see how our denial could be misleading us. In groups we learn to accept our place without grandiosity. We are just a single person, in some ways so different, yet in basic ways no different, from all of the others. It's a true lesson in humility. We may be models for other group members, while at the same time we see them as models for ourselves.

Groups can provide hope. We come to know others who grow and change. We hear what difficult times they have had, and we see them become spiritually healthy. We begin to see that our own circumstances, no matter how hard, can be dealt with, perhaps even turned into spiritually enriching experiences. Groups can be a wonderful support for the Eleventh Step. When we join together, we can make a kind of collective "conscious contact" with our individual Higher Powers. We consciously contact others with chronic illness or disability as we search for spiritual growth, and then we reinforce each other's "conscious contact" with his or her Higher Power.

This last requirement of Step Twelve asks that we live all we have learned. It suggests that when we have a problem or a concern, we review program principles, apply them to our current situation, and "practice them in all our affairs." If we consistently practice what we have learned, we will finally become what we practice.

Once a well-known New York psychiatrist visited a Hopi Indian reservation. He was fascinated by the Indian mind, and he thought that perhaps studying it would help his work. One day he was watching an old man weaving. The old man asked the psychiatrist what he did in the place he came from. The psychiatrist tried to explain that he worked with people's minds. The Hopi asked what that meant and the psychiatrist said that it was pretty complicated to explain, but it had to do with people whose feelings and emotions didn't function right. The old man asked if the psychiatrist could heal these people. The psychiatrist said that depended on the diagnosis. The Hopi then commented that all healing was in the dance, the dance of life. Intrigued by the idea, the psychiatrist asked if the old man would teach him the dance of life. And the Hopi said, "Yes, of course. But if you are going to dance, you have to move. You can't just watch, or listen, to it. I know it; you have to do it. I will teach you the steps, but you must bring your own music" (Carl Hammerschlag, *The Dancing Healers*).

If we who are chronically ill and disabled carry the music of the Twelve Step program, we can be healed as we go through the dance of life.

Step Twelve: Written Exercise

1. How can a spiritual awakening affect your life?
2. Describe how the spiritual changes you've already experienced have affected the way you think and feel.
3. What is one way you plan to carry the message of the Twelve Steps to others with chronic illness or disability? How can this help them? How can this help you?
4. What could you gain from belonging to a group of others with chronic illness or disability?

Step Twelve: Imagery Exercise

Imagine yourself sitting comfortably in a group with several other people who are chronically ill or disabled. You are relaxed, pleased to be there.

Imagine that you have decided to tell the group about

your condition, about all of the emotional pain you have felt. As you talk, describe not only the pain but also some of the things you have done as a result.

Explain how the Twelve Steps have helped you in the ways your life has changed. Also describe what parts of the Twelve Steps have seemed easy and with what parts you continue to struggle.

Talk a little about what you see as your challenge to spiritual growth in the future.

When you have finished, ask if any of the others would like to respond. If they do, listen to what they say. Don't argue; just hear them. Then thank them for giving you feedback and for listening to your story.

Now imagine yourself in a circle with the others, holding hands and repeating the Serenity Prayer.

God, grant me the serenity
To accept the things I cannot change,
The courage to change the things I can,
And the wisdom to know the difference.

Now return to your day, knowing that, whenever you choose, you can bring this image to life.

CHAPTER FOURTEEN

What Will Happen

As we live the Twelve Steps, what happens is awesome. Our illness or disability becomes a take-off point in our lives, rather than a dead end. We find the beginning of a new self, a new life, a new sense of time. In the past, we were imprisoned by our view of ourselves as ill or disabled "for the rest of our lives." Now we are freed from this constraint. We know that the rest of our lives can be lived one Step, one day at a time. It is the fulfillment of the moment that matters, not what has been or will someday be.

All humans go through life on a tightrope. Some of us are forced by circumstances to look down, and we are not the same as those who don't. We know, deep in our soul, the potential for vulnerability and catastrophe. For us, that potential has become real. Our chronic illness or disability has come to us, and we know that it won't disappear. But we have found another way. We have found a way to live so that our spiritual growth becomes more important to us than our concern with chronic physical problems and emotional pain.

Many philosophers tell us that the growth of the spirit is the ultimate goal of human existence. It isn't the evolution of our bodies, or the extent of our accomplishment or material success that matters, but the growth of our soul—our spirituality. Chronically ill and disabled people are put in a position where we may have to look beyond our physical being for fulfillment, because our physical being is limited. But there can be no limitations on the growth of our soul, and the Twelve Steps can guide us. The beauty of this program is that it can work for anyone. It provides a way to accept the truth of a Higher Power without binding it to dogma. It loosens the boundaries of what is spiritual and therefore can embrace people of all religious and philosophical beliefs.

There are some specific goals we strive for on our journey toward spiritual fulfillment. We strive to receive strength and understanding from the spiritual resources that surround us. We strive to surrender our self-centeredness and to practice honesty, humility, appreciation, and forgiveness. We strive to give service to others. And finally, we strive for balance.

We work toward balance between our involvement with the process we live and surrendering the outcome of that process. We are constantly trying to distinguish between willfully taking control of our lives and being appropriately responsible for them. Too often we try to force the balance in our lives, rather than simply allowing ourselves room for balance. We need to stay calm, to take it slowly, to quiet ourselves. Then we can find our center of balance, which leads us to peace, serenity, and joy. As ballet dancers and Yoga masters need balance in their spirits to move their bodies in unbelievable ways, so our spirit needs balance to be fulfilled.

Accept the Twelve Step program as a way of life and

we'll live happily ever after, right? If only it were that simple. When we accept the Steps as our basis for living, we must *work* them for the rest of our lives. On one hand, it gets even harder because we become increasingly aware of ourselves, of the world around us, and of what our responses need to be. On the other hand, it gets easier as our new ways become more habitual and as we become more deeply aware of the support our personal spiritual resources give us.

The Serenity Prayer (which some of us call the Serenity Meditation) can help. First, it teaches us that some things in our lives are beyond our control and some are even beyond our influence. Acceptance of the things we cannot change can lead us to serenity and open the door to a celebration of life.

Second, we receive the courage, dedication, and strength to take the responsibility for influencing those things that are not beyond our control—to change what we can. Both behavioral and spiritual change take much strength and much courage. We have learned that while we cannot change our physical condition, we can change our attitude toward our bodies and the way we live our lives. We have looked at our emotional pain and found that a new spiritual approach can help us turn the negatives of anger, jealousy, and fear into positive, creative energy. In the past, we may have anticipated change with fear and dread, which blocked our going forward. Now we are learning that change offers the opportunity to focus on our spirituality and gives us a chance to become more than we have ever been.

Finally, we are beginning to understand the difference between what we can change and what we cannot. Listening closely to the voice of our Higher Power helps us differentiate between the two. With our Higher Power's help, we can use all we know to stay with reality, to fight off the denial and rationalization that supports our past ways. In addition to the Serenity Prayer, there are other thoughts we use. We strive to do the following.

Surrender the outcome. Picture a spider web: small, delicate yet strong, spun across the corner of a kitchen baseboard. It's hardly noticeable, but a drama is taking place there that is important for us to watch. A small, unsuspecting fly flits near the web, veers too close, and gets caught. As the fly struggles, the spider, which has left the web to crawl across the kitchen floor, begins to scurry back to eat its victim. But a Siamese cat, blue eyes flashing, sable tail twitching, stalks the spider. As the cat is about to pounce on his tasty snack, a woman steps into the corner, crushing the spider and tearing down the web. The cat sits back on his haunches, staring at the woman. A small drama, almost meaningless. Or is it? What can this tiny incident teach us about control, about outcomes? The fly had no way of knowing that it would be caught in a web. The spider had no way of knowing that it was being stalked by a cat. The cat had no way of knowing that his mistress would destroy his treat. This is true for all of us, all of the time. We have no way of knowing. But we worry, and we fret, and we try to control outcomes, using precious energy. The fly, the spider, and the cat certainly didn't seem concerned about the outcomes in their lives, and it wouldn't have mattered if they had been. They had no control, and ultimately, neither do we. We need to surrender the outcome, to stop worrying, and to use our energy to be the very best we can for the moment that we have.

We can do our utmost to concentrate on each moment and whatever task or event is at hand. We can approach the moments of our lives with love and openness to their potential. We can live in the present, not in the past or the future. We can do this when we trust where the process is taking us, believing that wherever our lives go we will have the opportunity for spiritual growth. We can, with serenity, surrender the outcome. As a result, we drop our anxiety about the past and the future and concentrate on our moment in life. And that's really all there is—the rest is nonreality. What has been, was; what will be, is not yet.

Have the will for loving. We've learned that love isn't just romance or sex. We've learned that loving is to extend ourselves to nurture our own or another's spiritual growth. This means that life can be full of love—for ourselves, for our intimate friends and family, and for many other people whose paths we cross. We love ourselves when we are soft with ourselves, when we take time out to rest and reflect, when we treat ourselves to a new sweater or a movie, a trip, or a special time with a friend. We love ourselves when we are tough with ourselves too. We love ourselves when we don't let ourselves get caught in our old pain, when we force ourselves to attend to the new things we know, even though it would be so much easier to lapse back. We love ourselves when we focus our anger realistically, when we push ourselves to confront a fearful situation, and when we stand up for ourselves with our doctor, or boss, or loved one.

We can love others by hugging them and telling them they're terrific. We also love them when we confront them with their self-destructive behavior or about a problem in the relationship between us. At these times, we love them even though what we do makes them angry or they reject us. Our love shows in the process, not the outcome.

Love takes willpower, patience, attention, concentration, kindness, thoughtfulness, understanding, empathy, and toughness. Loving is hard; it takes so much energy, so much time. But loving is easier when we know that we are loved, that there are forces greater than ourselves that unfailingly support us. As this sense of love grows in our lives, we can share it with others. We have a model of being loved which we, in turn, can use to nurture those around us.

Stay open to the possibilities in each moment of our day. Until now, most of us have never done this. Even though we understand the individual words, it may be a hard idea to comprehend. Each moment of every day contains a myriad of possibilities. Each moment connects the past and the future. It brings the experience and knowledge acquired in the past into the present so we can make choices that will influence our future. What life really comes down to is choice. No matter what happens to us, as long as we are in a physically conscious state we retain the power of choice.

We can choose to recognize a Power greater than ourselves or we can choose to go it alone. We can choose to accept grace or to ignore its existence. We can choose to struggle toward perfection or to accept our human limitations. We have a choice of what to perceive, what decisions to make, what thoughts to think about what is happening, what feelings to have, and each choice will lead to a different outcome.

Take this moment as an example. You can choose to continue to read this book and to accept what it's saying about the importance and potential of each moment. You can feel excited about the prospect of enlarging your awareness in this way. This attitude may lead to behaviors that can broaden your life and experience. Or you can choose to be skeptical, saying, "Well, I don't know about this, but I'll think about it." Or you can choose to close the book, saying, "This is a bunch of junk." Each of these responses will lead to a different outcome. But whether we choose to close the book, question it, or believe its message, the reality is that this moment is all we have of life. We mentally recycle the past, holding on to its problems and its pain; we fantasize about the future, dreaming outcomes based on fear or desire, but we can only live the moment we are in.

An old saying goes "We only live for an instant, so make the best of it." This is generally understood to mean that within the greater scheme of things our individual life is very short, so we better live as well as we can. But it can also mean that there is no past and no future, only the instant, that moment when life happens. This instant is the only time we have to think, to feel, to act, and to choose. The exciting part is that each moment is a cross-roads, full of potential for growth, change, or stagnation. We need only stay open to the possibilities that it presents. Also, when life is hard, when we don't know how we can stand to go on, it helps to know that each instant in which we live is very short, that we can certainly handle this one tiny space of time.

Be present for the acceptance of joy or peace, and of grace or enlightenment. It's as if we are a jigsaw puzzle. We began the Twelve Steps with pieces of ourselves lying around, mixed up, some even upside down. We slowly began to arrange the pieces, beginning with the edges. We filled ourselves in, and our picture took shape. Finally, we are left with only one piece to drop in, just one, in the very center of our puzzle. We pick it up and fit it in. This is the piece that lives at our core. "Grace" is the Christian word for it; others call it "Enlightenment," still others, "Joy or Peace." The name doesn't matter. It is the powerful force that originates outside of human consciousness and that supports and protects and enhances the spiritual growth of human beings. This central piece contains the light that we carry within us. We can never control how dark it may get on the outside, but with this final part of ourselves in place, our inner light will always show us the way.

There is a Sanskrit greeting that folds all of this into one beautiful word. Translated, the greeting means "The light that shines within me salutes the light that shines within you." The word is "Namasté."

Appendixes

The Twelve Steps of Alcoholics Anonymous[*]

1. We admitted we were powerless over alcohol—that our lives had become unmanageable.
2. Came to believe that a Power greater than ourselves could restore us to sanity.
3. Made a decision to turn our will and our lives over to the care of God *as we understood Him.*
4. Made a searching and fearless moral inventory of ourselves.
5. Admitted to God, to ourselves, and to another human being the exact nature of our wrongs.
6. Were entirely ready to have God remove all these defects of character.
7. Humbly asked Him to remove our shortcomings.
8. Made a list of all persons we had harmed, and became willing to make amends to them all.
9. Made direct amends to such people wherever possible, except when to do so would injure them or others.
10. Continued to take personal inventory and when we were wrong promptly admitted it.

---

[*] The Twelve Steps are taken from *Alcoholics Anonymous,* 3d ed., published by AA World Services, Inc., New York, N.Y., pp. 59–60. Reprinted with permission. See editor's note on copyright page.

11. Sought through prayer and meditation to improve our conscious contact with God *as we understood Him,* praying only for knowledge of His will for us and the power to carry that out.

12. Having had a spiritual awakening as the result of these steps, we tried to carry this message to alcoholics, and to practice these principles in all our affairs.

The Twelve Steps for Chronically Ill or Disabled People*

1. We admitted we were powerless over our chronic illness or disability—that our lives had become unmanageable.
2. Came to believe that a Power greater than ourselves could restore us to sanity.
3. Made a decision to turn our will and our lives over to the care of the God of our understanding.
4. Made a searching and fearless moral inventory of ourselves.
5. Admitted to the God of our understanding, to ourselves, and to another human being the exact nature of our wrongs.
6. Were entirely ready to have the God of our understanding remove all of our defects of character.
7. Humbly asked God to remove our shortcomings.
8. Made a list of all persons we had harmed, and became willing to make amends to them all.
9. Made direct amends to such people wherever possible, except when to do so would injure them or others.

* Adapted from the Twelve Steps of Alcoholics Anonymous with permission of AA World Services, Inc., New York, N.Y.

Appendix B

10. Continued to take personal inventory and when we were wrong promptly admitted it.
11. Sought through prayer and meditation to improve our conscious contact with the God of our understanding, praying only for knowledge of God's will for us and the power to carry that out.
12. Having had a spiritual awakening as the result of these steps, we tried to carry this message to others with chronic illness or disability, and to practice these principles in all our affairs.

Serenity Prayer

God, grant me the serenity
To accept the things I cannot change,
The courage to change the things I can,
And the wisdom to know the difference.

Daily Meditations[*]

TODAY:

I will look at myself and realize that I have emotional pain that has become dominant in my life. I am at the mercy of my pain and unable to manage it. Understanding this, I admit that I need help.

I will acknowledge the presence of spiritual resources greater than myself that are fully capable of supporting me and healing my pain.

I will let go of my need to be physically "normal" and will focus instead on my spiritual growth. I will realize that my spiritual wellness can supersede my physical problems, that spiritual growth is the ultimate goal of humankind.

I will let go of my inclination to analyze and question my situation. I will surrender myself to live by the tenets of the Twelve Step recovery program. While I will continue to make my own life happen, I will accept that it is a Power greater than myself that shows me the way.

---

[*] Adapted with permission from *Twelve Steps for Adult Children*. San Diego: Recovery Publications, 1987.

I will release the past, forgiving myself and others for the ways we have been. Searching for fault, or blaming myself and others, keeps me stuck in the past.

I will drop my anxiety about the future. I will live this day with as much joy, trust, and serenity as I can, realizing that this day is all that I can handle.

I will concentrate on staying present in each moment, knowing that it is the only time I really have, the only time that I can effect change and growth in my life, the only time I can act toward my spiritual wellness.

I will take responsibility for all aspects of my life: my choices, my behavior, my feelings, my physical and mental health, my spiritual well-being, and the principles and values by which I live.

I will consciously use all my energies that contribute to the betterment of my life and the lives of others, such as expressing kindness, honesty, and integrity.

I will replace my negative thoughts with positive thoughts, knowing that positive thoughts lead to my spiritual growth.

I will be grateful for the opportunity to be set free from old attitudes and behaviors that prevent me from moving toward spiritual healing.

I will fully accept myself, just as I am, loving myself and realizing my value and worthiness to others.

I will go forth into this day with enthusiasm and with the determination to enjoy it and give it my positive best, come what may.

APPENDIX E

Finding a Mutual Aid Group

The groups that we generally call self-help groups are probably better called groups for mutual aid. Their underlying principle is that people help themselves by helping each other, and that the helper gets as much from the giving as the person who is helped.

Finding a mutual aid group is not difficult. The American Self-Help Clearinghouse helps both the general public and professionals to find and form no-fee mutual help support groups and networks for almost any type of emotional problem—illness, disability, addiction, loss, parenting, abuse, and other stressful life problems. You can access a search engine by logging onto: www.cmhc.com/selfhelp. Here you can learn about more than eight hundred national, international, and "model" self-help groups. You may also purchase the *Self-Help Sourcebook*, which is a guide that has been developed to act as a starting point for exploring real-life support groups in your community. Call the American Self-Help Clearinghouse by phone weekdays at 973-625-3037; TTY 625-9053.

Bibliography

Anderson, Daniel J. *Living with a Chronic Illness*. Center City, Minn.: Hazelden, 1986. Out of print.

Burnett, Frances. *The Secret Garden*. New York: Lippincott, J. B. Junior Books, 1962.

E., Stephanie. *Shame Faced: The Road to Recovery*. Center City, Minn.: Hazelden, 1986.

Hammerschlag, Carl. *The Dancing Healers*. New York: Harper and Row, 1989.

Kübler-Ross, Elisabeth. *On Death and Dying*. New York: Macmillan, 1969.

Little Red Book, The. Center City, Minn.: Hazelden, 1970.

Muller, Wayne. *How, Then, Shall We Live? Four Simple Questions That Reveal the Beauty and Meaning in Our Lives*. New York: Bantam Books, 1996.

Peck, M. Scott. *The Road Less Traveled: A New Psychology of Love, Traditional Values and Spiritual Growth*. New York: Simon and Schuster, 1978.

Rossi, Ernest Lawrence. *The Psychobiology of Mind-Body Healing: New Concepts of Therapeutic Hypnosis*. New York: W. W. Norton, 1986.

Siegel, Bernie. *Love, Medicine, and Miracles: Lessons Learned About Self-Healing from a Surgeon's Experience with Exceptional Patients.* New York: Harper and Row, 1986.

Touchstones: A Book of Daily Meditations for Men. Center City, Minn.: Hazelden, 1986.

Viorst, Judith. *Necessary Losses: The Loves, Illusions, Dependencies, and Impossible Expectations That All of Us Have to Give Up in Order to Grow.* New York: Ballantine Books, 1986.

Index

About the Author

MARTHA CLEVELAND's chronic illness proved to be one of the great gifts of her life. From it, she has learned that none of us has ultimate control over our own body, but we do have control over how we respond to whatever situation life hands us.

In her mid-thirties, her symptoms forced her into panic and despair, but over time, she has learned to accept her condition and live in a rich, wonderfully rewarding way. She went to the University of Minnesota, gained a bachelor's degree, a master's degree, and in 1978, a doctorate degree. She became a licensed consulting psychologist, working in private practice, an adjunct staff member with the Family Therapy Institute of Saint Paul, and a consultant to various agencies.

In her late sixties, she retired and is now living what she feels is the richest, most satisfying part of her life. She and her husband, Walter, live in the suburban home they bought forty-eight years ago. She is deeply involved with her family, friends, gardening, and the rescue work she does with retired racing greyhounds. She comes to this late part of her life knowing that it isn't circumstance that defines us; it is how we respond to that circumstance that will ultimately tell us who we are.

HAZELDEN INFORMATION AND EDUCATIONAL SERVICES is a division of the Hazelden Foundation, a not-for-profit organization. Since 1949, Hazelden has been a leader in promoting the dignity and treatment of people afflicted with the disease of chemical dependency.

The mission of the foundation is to improve the quality of life for individuals, families, and communities by providing a national continuum of information, education, and recovery services that are widely accessible; to advance the field through research and training; and to improve our quality and effectiveness through continuous improvement and innovation.

Stemming from that, the mission of this division is to provide quality information and support to people wherever they may be in their personal journey—from education and early intervention, through treatment and recovery, to personal and spiritual growth.

Although our treatment programs do not necessarily use everything Hazelden publishes, our bibliotherapeutic materials support our mission and the Twelve Step philosophy upon which it is based. We encourage your comments and feedback.

The headquarters of the Hazelden Foundation is in Center City, Minnesota. Additional treatment facilities are located in Chicago, Illinois; New York, New York; Plymouth, Minnesota; St. Paul, Minnesota; and West Palm Beach, Florida. At these sites, we provide a continuum of care for men and women of all ages. Our Plymouth facility is designed specifically for youth and families.

For more information on Hazelden, please call **1-800-257-7800**. Or you may access our World Wide Web site on the Internet at **www.hazelden.org**.